Superantigen Protocols

METHODS IN MOLECULAR BIOLOGY™

John M. Walker, Series Editor

225. **Inflammation Protocols,** edited by *Paul G. Winyard and Derek A. Willoughby, 2003*

224. **Functional Genomics:** *Methods and Protocols,* edited by *Michael J. Brownstein and Arkady Khodursky, 2003*

223. **Tumor Suppressor Genes:** *Volume 2: Regulation, Function, and Medicinal Applications,* edited by *Wafik S. El-Deiry, 2003*

222. **Tumor Suppressor Genes:** *Volume 1: Pathways and Isolation Strategies,* edited by *Wafik S. El-Deiry, 2003*

221. **Generation of cDNA Libraries:** *Methods and Protocols,* edited by *Shao-Yao Ying, 2003*

220. **Cancer Cytogenetics:** *Methods and Protocols,* edited by *John Swansbury, 2003*

219. **Cardiac Cell and Gene Transfer:** *Principles, Protocols, and Applications,* edited by *Joseph M. Metzger, 2003*

218. **Cancer Cell Signaling:** *Methods and Protocols,* edited by *David M. Terrian, 2003*

217. **Neurogenetics:** *Methods and Protocols,* edited by *Nicholas T. Potter, 2003*

216. **PCR Detection of Microbial Pathogens:** *Methods and Protocols,* edited by *Konrad Sachse and Joachim Frey, 2003*

215. **Cytokines and Colony Stimulating Factors:** *Methods and Protocols,* edited by *Dieter Körholz and Wieland Kiess, 2003*

214. **Superantigen Protocols,** edited by *Teresa Krakauer, 2003*

213. **Capillary Electrophoresis of Carbohydrates,** edited by *Pierre Thibault and Susumu Honda, 2003*

212. **Single Nucleotide Polymorphisms:** *Methods and Protocols,* edited by *Pui-Yan Kwok, 2003*

211. **Protein Sequencing Protocols, 2nd ed.,** edited by *Bryan John Smith, 2003*

210. **MHC Protocols,** edited by *Stephen H. Powis and Robert W. Vaughan, 2003*

209. **Transgenic Mouse Methods and Protocols,** edited by *Marten Hofker and Jan van Deursen, 2003*

208. **Peptide Nucleic Acids:** *Methods and Protocols,* edited by *Peter E. Nielsen, 2002*

207. **Recombinant Antibodies for Cancer Therapy:** *Methods and Protocols.* edited by *Martin Welschof and Jürgen Krauss, 2002*

206. **Endothelin Protocols,** edited by *Janet J. Maguire and Anthony P. Davenport, 2002*

205. ***E. coli* Gene Expression Protocols,** edited by *Peter E. Vaillancourt, 2002*

204. **Molecular Cytogenetics:** *Protocols and Applications,* edited by *Yao-Shan Fan, 2002*

203. ***In Situ* Detection of DNA Damage:** *Methods and Protocols,* edited by *Vladimir V. Didenko, 2002*

202. **Thyroid Hormone Receptors:** *Methods and Protocols,* edited by *Aria Baniahmad, 2002*

201. **Combinatorial Library Methods and Protocols,** edited by *Lisa B. English, 2002*

200. **DNA Methylation Protocols,** edited by *Ken I. Mills and Bernie H, Ramsahoye, 2002*

199. **Liposome Methods and Protocols,** edited by *Subhash C. Basu and Manju Basu, 2002*

198. **Neural Stem Cells:** *Methods and Protocols,* edited by *Tanja Zigova, Juan R. Sanchez-Ramos, and Paul R. Sanberg, 2002*

197. **Mitochondrial DNA:** *Methods and Protocols,* edited by *William C. Copeland, 2002*

196. **Oxidants and Antioxidants:** *Ultrastructure and Molecular Biology Protocols,* edited by *Donald Armstrong, 2002*

195. **Quantitative Trait Loci:** *Methods and Protocols,* edited by *Nicola J. Camp and Angela Cox, 2002*

194. **Posttranslational Modifications of Proteins:** *Tools for Functional Proteomics,* edited by *Christoph Kannicht, 2002*

193. **RT-PCR Protocols,** edited by *Joe O'Connell, 2002*

192. **PCR Cloning Protocols, 2nd ed.,** edited by *Bing-Yuan Chen and Harry W. Janes, 2002*

191. **Telomeres and Telomerase:** *Methods and Protocols,* edited by *John A. Double and Michael J. Thompson, 2002*

190. **High Throughput Screening:** *Methods and Protocols,* edited by *William P. Janzen, 2002*

189. **GTPase Protocols:** *The RAS Superfamily,* edited by *Edward J. Manser and Thomas Leung, 2002*

188. **Epithelial Cell Culture Protocols,** edited by *Clare Wise, 2002*

187. **PCR Mutation Detection Protocols,** edited by *Bimal D. M. Theophilus and Ralph Rapley, 2002*

186. **Oxidative Stress Biomarkers and Antioxidant Protocols,** edited by *Donald Armstrong, 2002*

185. **Embryonic Stem Cells:** *Methods and Protocols,* edited by *Kursad Turksen, 2002*

184. **Biostatistical Methods,** edited by *Stephen W. Looney, 2002*

183. **Green Fluorescent Protein:** *Applications and Protocols,* edited by *Barry W. Hicks, 2002*

182. ***In Vitro* Mutagenesis Protocols, 2nd ed.,** edited by *Jeff Braman, 2002*

181. **Genomic Imprinting:** *Methods and Protocols,* edited by *Andrew Ward, 2002*

180. **Transgenesis Techniques, 2nd ed.:** *Principles and Protocols,* edited by *Alan R. Clarke, 2002*

179. **Gene Probes:** *Principles and Protocols,* edited by *Marilena Aquino de Muro and Ralph Rapley, 2002*

178. **Antibody Phage Display:** *Methods and Protocols,* edited by *Philippa M. O'Brien and Robert Aitken, 2001*

177. **Two-Hybrid Systems:** *Methods and Protocols,* edited by *Paul N. MacDonald, 2001*

176. **Steroid Receptor Methods:** *Protocols and Assays,* edited by *Benjamin A. Lieberman, 2001*

175. **Genomics Protocols,** edited by *Michael P. Starkey and Ramnath Elaswarapu, 2001*

174. **Epstein-Barr Virus Protocols,** edited by *Joanna B. Wilson and Gerhard H. W. May, 2001*

173. **Calcium-Binding Protein Protocols, Volume 2:** *Methods and Techniques,* edited by *Hans J. Vogel, 2001*

172. **Calcium-Binding Protein Protocols, Volume 1:** *Reviews and Case Histories,* edited by *Hans J. Vogel, 2001*

171. **Proteoglycan Protocols,** edited by *Renato V. Iozzo, 2001*

170. **DNA Arrays:** *Methods and Protocols,* edited by *Jang B. Rampal, 2001*

169. **Neurotrophin Protocols,** edited by *Robert A. Rush, 2001*

168. **Protein Structure, Stability, and Folding,** edited by *Kenneth P. Murphy, 2001*

METHODS IN MOLECULAR BIOLOGY™

Superantigen Protocols

Edited by

Teresa Krakauer

Uniformed Services University of the Health Sciences, Bethesda, MD
US Army Medical Research Institute of Infectious Diseases,
Frederick, MD

Humana Press ✳ **Totowa, New Jersey**

Cover design by Patricia F. Cleary.
Cover illustration: From Fig. 3B in Chapter 5 by S. Munir Alam and Nicholas R. J. Gascoigne; from Fig. 2 in Chapter 11 by Teresa Krakauer, Xin Chen, O. M. Zack Howard, and Howard A. Young; and from Fig. 2 in Chapter 12 by Lars Björk.

Production Editor: Kim Hoather-Potter.

For additional copies, pricing for bulk purchases, and/or information about other Humana titles, contact Humana at the above address or at any of the following numbers: Tel: 973-256-1699; Fax: 973-256-8341; E-mail: humana@humanapr.com, or visit our Website at www.humanapress.com

Library of Congress Cataloging in Publication Data

Main entry under title: Methods in molecular biology™.

Superantigen protocols/edited by Teresa Krakauer
    p.;cm.--(Methods in molecular biology; 214)
    Includes bibliographical references and index.
    ISBN 0-89603-984-6 (alk. paper)
    1. Superantigens--Laboratory manuals.
    [DNLM: 1. Superantigens. 2. Clinical Laboratory Techniques. QW 573
    S958 2002] I. Krakauer, Teresa. II. Methods in molecular biology
    (Clifton, N.J.); v. 214.
        QR186.6.S94 S867 2002
        616.07'92--dc21   2002017291

Dedication

To my super-family for providing me with an enriched environment to study and learn.

Teresa Krakauer, PhD

Preface

Superantigen Protocols assembles experimental protocols that have proved useful for the study of superantigens. These techniques will allow researchers from various areas of cell biology, microbiology, immunology, biochemistry, and molecular biology to assess the physical characteristics and biological effects of well-known superantigens as well as of putative substances that might have superantigenic activities, and to explore therapies for superantigen-induced effects.

Microbial exotoxins have been studied for decades as virulence factors because of their pathogenic effects. The term "superantigen" was coined by Marrack and Kappler a decade ago for some of these molecules because of their potent T-cell stimulatory activities. In recent years, advances in molecular biology provide recombinant as well as natural superantigens in highly purified form for physical characterization. Superantigens are now used extensively as tools to study interactions between receptors on cells of the immune system as they bind to major histocompatibility complex class II molecules on antigen-presenting cells and V_β regions of T-cell receptors. The biological effects that result from these interactions are studied both in vitro and in vivo. The intent of this book is, therefore, to bring together up-to-date techniques developed by experts in the field of biochemistry, immunology, and molecular biology for the study of superantigens.

Superantigen Protocols begins with an overview of the field to provide background information on the various classes of superantigens and their structure. This summary is followed by a group of chapters on methods to define binding and other physical interactions of superantigens with their cellular receptors. Finally, techniques used in the study of the biological effects of superantigens are covered to guide researchers in the assessment of cellular activities and molecules induced by superantigens. In addition, approaches to the study and the development of therapeutics in suppressing the superantigen-induced effects are presented.

Teresa Krakauer, PhD

Contents

Dedication v

Preface vii

Contributors...xi

1   Superantigens: *Structure, Function, and Diversity*
    Matthew D. Baker and K. Ravi Acharya *1*

2   Expression, Purification, and Detection of Novel Streptococcal
    Superantigens
    John K. McCormick and Patrick M. Schlievert *33*

3   Flow Cytometric Detection of MMTV Superantigens
    Gary Winslow *45*

4   Spectrophotometric Methods for the Determination
    of Superantigen Structure and Stability
    Anders Cavallin, Karin Petersson, and Göran Forsberg *55*

5   Binding Kinetics of Superantigen with TCR and MHC Class II
    S. Munir Alam and Nicholas R. J. Gascoigne *65*

6   Directed Evolution of T-Cell Receptors for Binding Superantigens
    Hywyn R. O. Churchill and David M. Kranz *87*

7   Analysis of Superantigen Binding to Soluble T-Cell Receptors
    Hywyn R. O. Churchill and David M. Kranz *101*

8   Role of Accessory Molecules in the Superantigen-Induced
    Activation of Peripheral Blood T Cells
    Catherine Gelin, Marie-Thérèse Zilber,
    and Dominique Charron *113*

9   T-Lymphocyte Activation Induced by Staphylococcal
    Enterotoxin Superantigens: *Analysis of Protein Tyrosine*
    Phosphorylation
    Anne Roumier, Florence Niedergang, and Andrés Alcover *127*

10 Measurement of Proinflammatory Cytokines and T-Cell
    Proliferative Response in Superantigen-Activated Human
    Peripheral Blood Mononuclear Cells
    Teresa Krakauer *137*

11 RNase Protection Assay for the Study of the Differential Effects
    of Therapeutic Agents in Suppressing Staphylococcal
    Enterotoxin B-Induced Cytokines in Human Peripheral
    Blood Mononuclear Cells
    Teresa Krakauer, Xin Chen, O. M. Zack Howard,
    and Howard A. Young 151

12 Staining Protocol for Superantigen-Induced Cytokine Production
    Studied at the Single-Cell Level
    Lars Björk 165

13 Assessment of Specific T-Cell Activation by Superantigens
    Natalie Sutkowski and Brigitte T. Huber 185

14 Superantigen-Induced Changes in Epithelial Ion Transport
    and Barrier Function: *Use of an In Vitro Model*
    James L. Watson and Derek M. McKay 219

15 Pyrogenic, Lethal, and Emetic Properties of Superantigens
    in Rabbits and Primates
    John K. McCormick, Gregory A. Bohach,
    and Patrick M. Schlievert 245

Index 255

Contributors

K. RAVI ACHARYA • *Department of Biology and Biochemistry, University of Bath, Claverton Down, Bath, UK*

S. MUNIR ALAM • *Division of Rheumatology, Allergy and Clinical Immunology, Department of Medicine, Duke University Medical Center, Durham, NC*

ANDRÉS ALCOVER • *Unité de Biologie des Interactions Cellulaires, Institut Pasteur, Paris, France*

MATTHEW D. BAKER • *Department of Biology and Biochemistry, University of Bath, Claverton Down, Bath, UK*

LARS BJÖRK • *Department of Biopharmaceutical Development, Biovitrum, Stockholm, Sweden*

GREGORY A. BOHACH • *Department of Microbiology, Molecular Biology and Biochemistry, University of Idaho, Moscow, ID*

ANDERS CAVALLIN • *Department of Molecular Biology, Astra Zeneca, Mölndel, Sweden*

DOMINIQUE CHARRON • *Inserm U396, Institut Biomedical des Cordeliers Université, Paris, France*

XIN CHEN • *Laboratory of Molecular Immunoregulation, National Cancer Institute, Frederick, MD*

HYWYN R. O. CHURCHILL • *Department of Biochemistry, University of Illinois, Urbana, IL*

GÖRAN FORSBERG • *Department of Biology, Active Biotech Research, Lund, Sweden*

NICHOLAS R. J. GASCOIGNE • *Department of Immunology, The Scripps Research Institute, La Jolla, CA*

CATHERINE GELIN • *Inserm U396, Inst d'Hématologie, Hôpital Saint-Louis, Paris, France*

O. M. ZACK HOWARD • *Laboratory of Molecular Immunoregulation, National Cancer Institute, Frederick, MD*

BRIGITTE T. HUBER • *Department of Pathology, Tufts University School of Medicine, Boston, MA*

TERESA KRAKAUER • *Department of Preventive Medicine and Biometrics, Uniformed Services University of the Health Sciences, Bethesda, MD; Department of Immunology and Molecular Biology, United States Army Medical Research Institute of Infectious Diseases, Fort Detrick, Frederick, MD*

xi

DAVID M. KRANZ • *Department of Biochemistry, University of Illinois, Urbana, IL*

JOHN K. MCCORMICK • *The Lawson Health Research Institute, and Department of Microbiology and Immunology, The University of Western Ontario, London, Ontario, Canada*

DEREK M. MCKAY • *Intestinal Disease Research Programme, McMaster University, Hamilton, Ontario, Canada*

FLORENCE NIEDERGANG • *Unité de Biologie des Interactions Cellulaires, Institut Pasteur, Paris, France*

KARIN PETERSSON • *Department of Biology, Active Biotech Research, Lund, Sweden*

ANNE ROUMIER • *Unité de Biologie des Interactions Cellulaires, Institut Pasteur, Paris, France*

PATRICK M. SCHLIEVERT • *Department of Microbiology, University of Minnesota Medical School, Minneapolis, MN*

NATALIE SUTKOWSKI • *Department of Pathology, Tufts University School of Medicine, Boston, MA*

JAMES L. WATSON • *Intestinal Disease Research Programme, McMaster University, Hamilton, Ontario, Canada*

GARY WINSLOW • *Wadsworth Center, New York State Department of Health, Albany, NY; Department of Biomedical Sciences, State University of New York at Albany, Albany, NY*

HOWARD A. YOUNG • *Laboratory of Experimental Immunology, National Cancer Institute, Frederick, MD*

MARIE-THÉRÈSE ZILBER • *Inserm U396, Inst d'Hématologie, Hôpital Saint-Louis, Paris, France*

1

Superantigens

Structure, Function, and Diversity

Matthew D. Baker and K. Ravi Acharya

1. Overview of Superantigens

Bacterial superantigens are potent T-cell stimulatory protein molecules produced by *Staphylococcus aureus* and *Streptococcus pyogenes (1)*. Their function in the microbe appears primarily to debilitate the host sufficiently through their effects on cells of the immune system to permit the causation of disease *(2)*. Their superantigenic activity can be attributed to their ability to bind to both major histocompatibility complex (MHC) class II molecules and T cell receptors by forming a trimolecular complex *(1)*. Unlike conventional antigens they are not processed internally by antigen presenting cells (APC), and are thus not displayed as peptide antigen in the peptide-binding groove of the MHC class II molecule. Superantigens bind to APCs on the outside of MHC class II molecule and to T cells *via* the external face of the T-cell receptor (TCR) V_β element (*see* **Fig. 1**). Each superantigen interacts with a specific V_β region of the TCR, stimulating a large fraction of T cells (for example, up to 10% of resting T cells) *(3)*.

From: *Methods in Molecular Biology, vol. 214: Superantigen Protocols*
Edited by: T. Krakauer © Humana Press Inc., Totowa, NJ

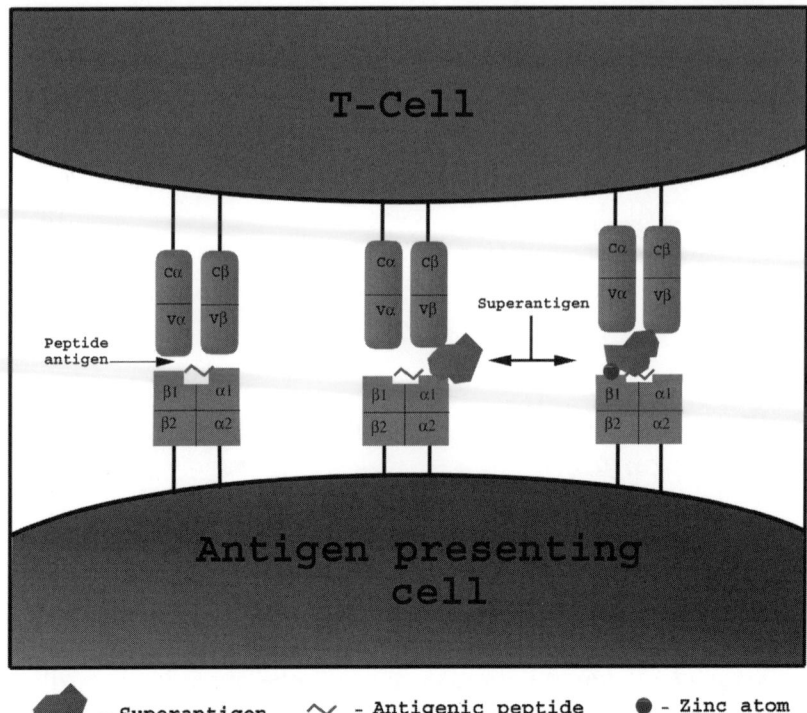

Fig. 1. Schematic representation illustrating the differences between conventional peptide antigen presentation and superantigen presentation to MHC class II and TCRs: Left to right, conventional antigen is processed by the APC and displayed as discrete peptide fragments within the peptide binding groove of MHC class II molecules. Interaction occurs between TCR and MHC class II molecule through two possible modes: 1) superantigens bind to the solvent exposed face of the MHC class II molecule ($\alpha 1$) *via* its generic site, forming a bridge between TCR (V_β) and MHC class II molecule; 2) Interaction also occurs between TCR V_α and MHC class II molecule involving the β-chain ($\beta 1$) where the superantigen binds to MHC class II molecule *via* a bridging zinc atom. In both cases the MHC class II-associated antigenic peptide has been shown to influence T-cell recognition of superantigen/MHC class II molecule complex.

Staphylococcal enterotoxins (SEs) A, B, C1-3, D, E, H; toxic shock syndrome toxin-1 (TSST-1); the streptococcal pyrogenic exotoxins (SPEs) A, C, H; streptococcal mitogenic exotoxin SMEZ-2 and streptococcal superantigen (SSA) are the most well studied superantigens to date (for recent reviews *see* Papageorgiou et al. *[4,5]*). Other pathogens, such as *Mycoplasma arthritidis* and *Yersinia enterocolitica*, have also been shown to secrete superantigenic proteins, though they are yet to be fully characterized *(6)*. Viral superantigens are implicated with infections caused by rabies virus, Epstein-Barr virus (EBV), and human herpesvirus, including HIV *(7,8)*. In this chapter we shall focus our discussion on bacterial superantigens.

2. Physical Characteristics of Superantigens

2.1. Common Architecture

The superantigen family comprises proteins of 22–29 kDa in size that are highly resistant to proteases and heat denaturation *(1)*. Based on amino acid sequence alignment of streptococcal and staphylococcal superantigens it is possible to divide them into three subfamilies: (1) SEA, SED, SEE, SEH, and SEI; (2) SEB, SEC1-3, SPEA1-3, SSA, and SEG and (3) SPEC, SPEJ, SPEG, SMEZ, and SMEZ-2. TSST-1 has ~28% homology with other SEs and cannot be grouped with any of these subfamilies. Comparison of the three-dimensional structures of superantigens (*see* Papageorgiou and Acharya *[4,5]* and references therein) reveals a conserved two-domain architecture (N- and C- terminal domains) and the presence of a long, solvent-accessible α-helix spanning the center of the molecule (*see* **Fig. 2**). The N-terminal domain has considerable structural similarity to the oligosaccharide/oligonucleotide-binding fold (OB-fold) found in other proteins of unrelated sequence, and is characterized by the presence of hydrophobic residues in its solvent-exposed regions. As its name implies, in other proteins the OB-fold is involved in DNA binding or carbohydrate recognition though no such activity has been attributed to superantigens so far. The C-terminal domain is composed of a four-stranded β-sheet capped by the central α-helix. Structurally, it is reminiscent of the β-grasp motif found in other proteins. Other common features include a highly flexible disulphide loop (*see* **Fig. 2**), present in the N-termi-

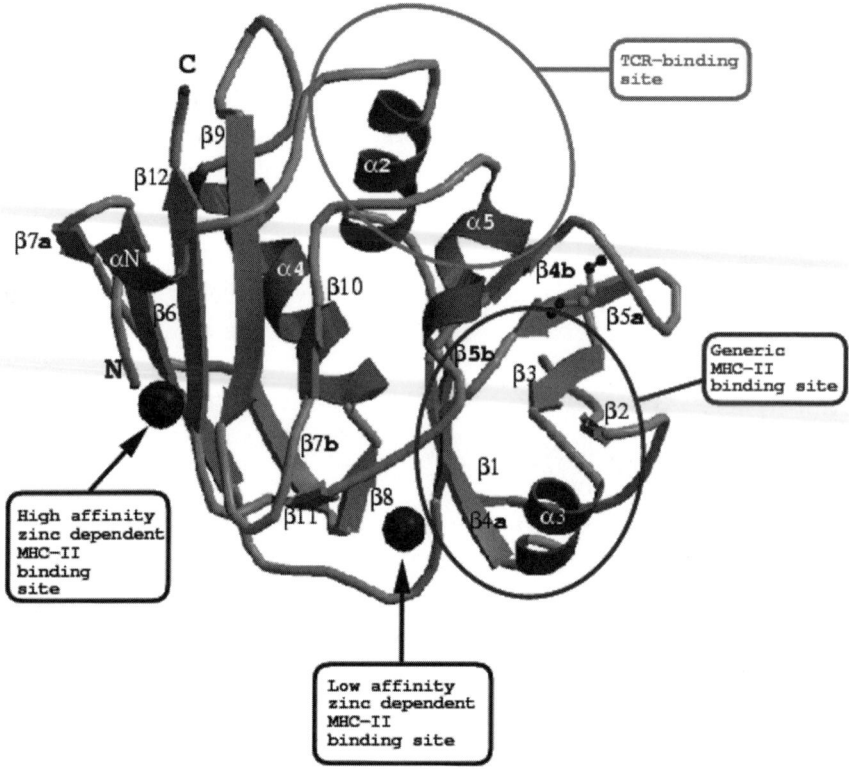

Fig. 2. Ribbon diagram of SEA representative of the common structural features of the superantigen family.

nal domain of SEs and SPEA, but not in TSST-1 and SPEC. This flexible loop is implicated in the emetic properties of the SEs and indeed mutation of the residues that form this disulphide loop to alanine abolishes the emetic activity in SEC1 *(9)*. Moreover mutation of either one of the cysteine residues in SPEA also reduces its ability to stimulate certain populations of T cells significantly *(10)*.

2.2. Purification Procedures

Several procedures have been adopted to purify superantigens in their native forms *(11–15)*. Most of them are multi-step procedures and are not always suitable for large-scale toxin production. Brehm et al. *(16)* developed a single-step dye ligand chromatography assay for the purification of SEA, SEB, SEC2, and TSST-1 using Red A gel. The procedure caters for both small- and large-scale preparations of toxins from *S. aureus* with good yields. Many studies have favored the use of recombinant toxins. These proteins can be produced as fusion proteins such as GST-tagged *(17,18)* or His-tagged toxins *(19)*, allowing a simple two-step cleavage and purification method. In all cases, whether native or recombinant, further purification by isoelectric focussing may be required to produce a single isoform. The exclusion of bioactive contaminants during toxin purification is esstential. For example, native SPEA, commercially available SPEA and recombinant SPEA preparations were all shown to be contaminated with DNase and an unknown protease. This contamination interferes with many immunological assays as DNase has been shown to independently induce cytokines *(20)*. A balance must be achieved therefore, between ease of purification and the purity of the final sample.

2.3. Detection Methods

There are several reliable assays for the detection of bacterial superantigens; namely the micro-slide, double-diffusion, and, enzyme-linked immunosorbent assay (ELISA)-based methods. Qualitative assays for bacterial superantigens are performed using the following technique *(21)*. Briefly, an agar plate cultured with the test organism has hyperimmune antisera and purified superantigen added to separate wells punched 4 mm to each other from the growing organism. After 12 h incubation at 37°C, the plate was examined for the formation of a precipitation arc that forms between antibodies present in the anti-sera and the superantigen, both in its purified form and from the cultured organism, if present. Quantitative assays such as the double immunodiffusion allow an estimate of the amount of toxin present in an isolate by comparison to an assay performed on a control toxin of known concentration. The detection range of this method, approx 4 µg/mL, can be extended two- to fourfold by drying and staining the slides *(21)*.

Several ELISA-based methods for the detection of superantigens have been developed *(22–24)* allowing multiple samples to be tested accurately and relatively quickly within a detection range of 0.03–0.05 μg/mL. Commercially available kits based on several of the above methods are available such as Ridascreen (R-Biopharm GmbH, Germany) and TECRA (International Bioproducts, Redmond, WA), which are ELISA kits for the detection of SEs A to E. A reversed passive latex agglutination assay kit, SET-RPLA (Oxoid, Ontario, Canada), can also be used for the detection of SEA, B, C, D, and E.

3. Biological Properties of Superantigens

3.1. Binding to MHC Class II Molecules

Structural analyses using X-ray crystallography have shown that MHC class II molecules possess two distinct superantigen binding sites (for details see Papageorgiou and Acharya *[4,5]*). The first, a low-affinity binding site (referred to as the generic site) is located on the α-chain of the MHC class II molecule and the second, a high-affinity (~100 times higher affinity than the generic site) zinc-dependent site is located on the β-chain (*see* **Fig. 3**). The structures of SEB and TSST-1 in complex with HLA-DR1 *via* the low affinity site *(25,30)*, SPEC in complex with HLA-DR2 *(26)* and SEH in complex with HLA-DR1 *(27) via* the high-affinity site have yielded a great deal of information about the binding of SAgs to MHC class II molecules. Each superantigen binds to different alleles of class II molecules to varying degrees. Whereas the majority of the superantigens including TSST-1 and SEB bind preferentially to HLA-DR alleles, superantigens such as SEC, SPEA, and SSA bind predominantly to HLA-DQ alleles *(18,28,29)*.

For both SEB and TSST-1 in complex with HLA-DR1, similar binding modes with the α-chain of DR1 involving the solvent-exposed, hydrophobic core at the N-terminal domain of the toxin molecule were evident. Similar hydrophobic ridge regions (except SPEC, SPEH, and SMEZ-2) form the generic site and are implicated in class II binding. However, in the case of TSST-1 additional

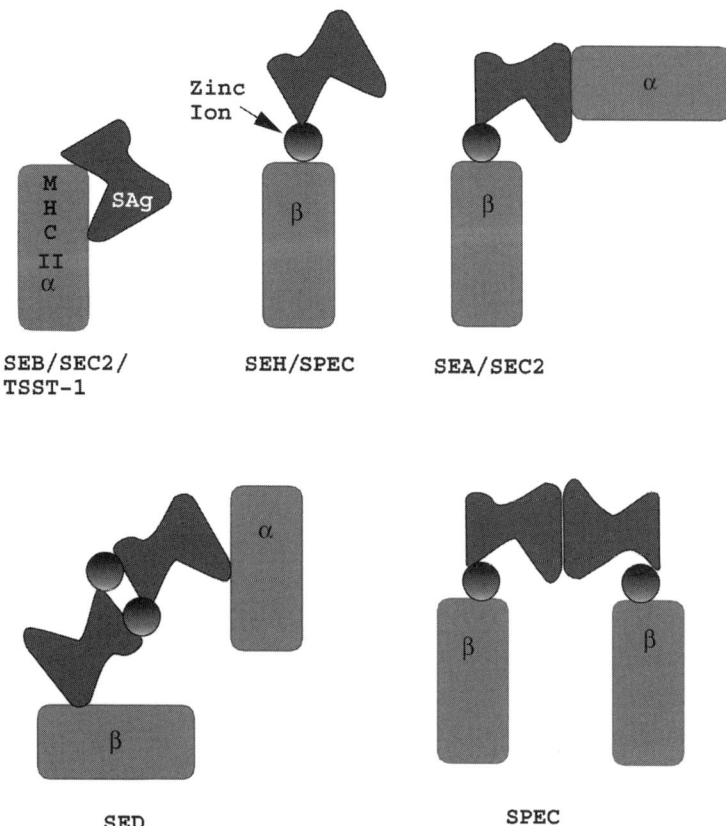

Fig. 3. Schematic diagram illustrating the multiple modes by which superantigens can interact with MHC class II molecules.

contacts with the peptide antigen were also present *(30)*. Indeed, truncating the C-terminal end of the peptide dramatically effects TSST-1 binding to murine I-Ab *(31)*.

In addition, several members of the superantigen family (except SEB, TSST-1, and SSA) possess either one or two zinc binding sites *(4)* (for details *see* **Table 1** and **Figs. 2** and **3**). The presence of the zinc ion is important for the recognition of class II molecules. Mutational and structural analyses have identified a high-affinity zinc-binding site in SEA at the C-terminal domain with a K_d of 100 nM for DR1 recognition *(32)*. However, the zinc-independent generic site at the N-terminal domain has considerably lower

Table 1
Comparison of the High-Affinity (Zinc-Dependent), and Low-Affinity (Generic) MHC Class II Binding Sites in Staphylococcal and Streptococcal Superantigens

Superantigen	MHC-II binding generic site	Zinc ligands	Reference
Staphylococcal			
SEA	Yes	High-affinity site S1, H187, H225, D227	(32,95)
		Low-affinity site D86, H114, E39$_{(mol2)}$, H$_2$O	
SEB	Yes	No	(96)
SEC2	Yes	H118, H122, D83, D9$_{(Symmetry\ related\ molecule)}$	(28)
SED	Yes	H218$_{(mol1)}$, D182$_{(mol2)}$, H220$_{(mol2)}$, D222$_{(mol2)}$[a]	
		Low-affinity site H8, E12, H109$_{(mol2)}$, K113$_{(mol2)}$	
SEE	Yes	H187, H225, D227	(35)
SEG		No	(32)
SEH	No generic site	H206, D208	(19)
SEI		No	(37)
TSST-1	Yes	No	(19)
			(97)
Streptococcal			
SPEA	Yes	E33, D77, H106, H110	(29,98,99)
SPEC	No generic site	H167, H201, D203	(26,36)
SPEG	No generic site	H167, H202, D204[b]	(17)
SPEH	No generic site	H198, D200, D160[b]	(17)
SMEZ	No generic site	H202, D204, H162[b]	(17)
SMEZ-2	No generic site	H202, D204, H162[b]	(17,100)
SMEZ3/SPEX	No generic site	H202, D204, H162[b]	(17,100)
SSA	Yes	No	(101)
			(18)

[a]And vice versa (mol1–mol2) for second zinc atom.

8

affinity (K_d of 10 μM) for class II binding. If the two binding sites co-exist, SEA shows a K_d of 13 nM. Mutations of residues in either of these sites results in a toxin unable to induce cytokine expression in peripheral blood mononuclear cells (PBMC) *(33)*. Thus in the case of SEA molecule, it possesses two distinct MHC class II binding sites, which might enable the formation of the trimeric SEA-MHC-SEA complex as observed in solution experiments *(34)* (*see* **Fig. 3**). Similar arguments can be put forward for SEE as both SEA and SEE possess identical zinc ligands.

In the case of SEC and SPEA, the high-affinity zinc-binding site observed in SEA is not present. However, a new zinc-binding site with somewhat lower affinity compared with the high-affinity zinc-binding described earlier (the estimated dissociation constant for the zinc ion in SEC2 is <1 μM) was identified at the N-terminal domain, which also appears to be important for MHC class II binding (*see* **Fig. 2**) *(29)*. We shall refer to this site as the secondary zinc-binding site. In SED *(35)* and SPEC *(36)*, the situation is slightly different since this toxin can form zinc-dependent homodimers (in SED) and zinc-independent homodimers (in SPEC) and binds solely to the β-chain of MHC class II molecule by a zinc-mediated mechanism similar to that of SEA and could form either trimers or tetramers. A similar binding mechanism has been proposed for SEH that also lacks a generic MHC class II binding site *(37)* (*see* **Fig. 3**).

The recent structures of SPEC in complex with HLA-DR2 *(26)* and SEH in complex with HLA-DR1 *(27)* *via* the high-affinity zinc-dependent site have shed more light on the interactions of superantigens with MHC class II molecules (*see* **Fig. 3**). The interaction between both superantigens and their MHC class II molecules is mediated by a bridging zinc ion, which tetrahedrally co-ordinates three ligands from the SPEC (His 167, His 201, and Asp 203) and two from SEH (His 206, Asp 208, and a water molecule) with one from the MHC class II β1 helix (His 81). There is also extensive contact between SPEC and the class II-associated antigenic peptide (approximately one-third of the contact surface area) and stabilization of the SEH-MHC class II complex also occurs through interaction with the antigenic peptide. Both the SPEC and SEH complexes have similar interactions with the antigenic peptide despite the fact that the peptides in each structure are different. This indicates that although the peptide plays an important role in the complex interaction, superantigen/MHC binding is not entirely peptide specific as a majority of the interactions with the peptide is with its backbone atoms.

Zinc is also shown to play a role in the binding of SMEZ-2, SPEG, and SPEH to MHC class II molecules, as the binding of all three of these superantigens to LG-2 cells is significantly reduced by the addition of EDTA *(17)*. The proposed zinc-binding site in each of these superantigens is shown to be closest to that of SEA and SPEC, both of which have geometrically and spatially equivalent sites *(17,36)*. As the presence of the zinc binding ligands suggest, all three of these superantigens bind to MHC class II molecules in a zinc-dependent fashion.

There appears to be a great deal of diversity in the mechanism by which superantigens can mediate with MHC class II molecules, either through zinc-mediated interaction or *via* the generic site or involving both site/s giving each superantigen a unique array of possible interactions through which it can exploit the immune system.

3.2. Binding to TCR-V$_\beta$ Regions

The characterization of superantigen-TCR binding region reveals many similarities and differences. This is reflected by the fact that they bind to TCR through a somewhat similar mechanism, yet have different V$_\beta$ specificities. The binding is mediated by interactions between the side-chains of the superantigen and the V$_\beta$ backbone atoms in a manner similar to that of MHC-peptide and antigen-antibody complexes *(38)*. The TCR binding site has been shown to involve a shallow cavity between the two domains of the molecule. For SEB this cavity is formed by residues 22–33 (mostly α2 helix), 55–61 (β2-β3 loop), 87–92 (β4 strand and β4-β5 loop), 112 (β5 strand) and 210–214 (α5 helix) *(39)* (*see* **Fig. 2**). Analogous sites for SEC and SEA have also been proposed. The crystal structures of

SEC2 and SEC3 in complex with TCR V_β chain by Fields et al. *(40)* has further elucidated the detailed interactions of superantigens with a TCR molecule. The main interactions are shown to be between the side-chain atoms of the superantigen and complementarity determining regions one and two (CDRs 1 and 2), and hypervariable region 4 (HV4) of the V_β chain. Comparison of this TCR binding site (from SEC2/3) with the corresponding regions of SEA and SEB identifies an invariant asparagine residue (Asn23 in SEB/SECs; Asn25 in SEA), as being crucial for direct interactions with the TCR. Mutation of this residue in SEB results in the loss of T-cell stimulation *(41)*. This residue is solvent exposed in SEA, SEB, and SEC, and is thought to be involved in similar interactions with the TCR in all the SEs. Leder et al. *(42)* evaluated the functional contribution of individual SEC3 residues to the stabilization of the SEC3/V_β complex by alanine scanning mutagenesis of all the residues of SEC3 shown to be in contact with the β-chain in the crystal structure *(40)*. It was found that the mutations that had the most effect on binding to the TCR-β-chain were Asn23, Tyr90, and Gln210. Tyr90 and Gln210 are conserved among SEC1-3, SEB, SPEA, and SSA has analogous residues Asn49, Tyr116, and Gln223 *(39)*. As mentioned earlier, the variance between superantigens with regard to TCR affinity and specificity can be accounted for by several residues unique to each particular superantigen as well as the any topological influence that each of these might have. For example, the residue Tyr26 of SEC2 confers specificity between SEC1 and SEC2 via its interaction with Gly53 from the V_β chain *(43)*. This residue is not conserved in SEA or SEB. Val91 of SEC2 is also implicated in TCR binding. This residue is not conserved in SEA (Tyr94) or SEB (Tyr91) either *(34)* and it is thought that the replacement of Val91 by a tyrosine residue in SEB may be responsible for its reduced affinity for the $V_\beta8.2$ chain *(40)*. Ser206, Asn207, and Thr21 have been identified as the probable specificity defining residues in SEA *(39)*. This is highlighted by the exchange of residues 206 and 207 in SEA for the homologous residues in SEE causing the profile of V_β elements on the responding T cells to change to that of SEE *(44)*.

Ser206 and Asn207 in SEA correspond to Gln210 and Ser211, respectively, in both SEB and SEC2. The greatest energetic contribution to the stability of the V_β-superantigen complex is made by those residues that define its specificity for particular V_β elements *(38)*.

The TCR binding site of TSST-1 is located in the C-terminal domain on the long $\alpha 2$ helix and between the $\beta 7$-$\beta 8$ and $\alpha 2$-$\beta 9$ loops as part of the $\alpha 1$ helix. In this regard, it is unique from the SEs *(45)*. Mitogenicity is lost either partially or completely, by mutation of residues in the region 115-144. Specifically, residues Tyr115, Glu132, His 135, Ile140, His 141, and Tyr144 were shown to be of major importance for TSST-1 binding to TCR *(45,46)*. Mutation of these residues produce substantially less mitogenic toxins, yet they can still be recognized by a specific antibody *(46)*. The TCR binding site of SPEC is as yet not fully characterized. As it is structurally very similar to TSST-1, it is possible that SPEC shares similar TCR binding characteristics.

In summary, the interactions between superantigens and TCR share a common core of residues with specificity for particular V_β elements being supplied by further residues unique to each toxin, giving rise to a characteristic V_β repertoire.

3.3. Signal Transduction Pathways of Superantigens

The primary targets of superantigens are the $CD4^+$ T cells *(47)*, activation of which results in T helper type 1 (Th1) cytokine release with no apparent Th2 response *(48)*. The consequences of a dominant Th1 response include suppression of antibody expression and reduced clearance of the invading microbe. A model of superantigen signal transduction can be constructed based on the TCR-oligomerization model of T-cell activation. This model proposes that binding of a ligand to TCR induces clustering of the TCRs on the cell surface, facilitating the recruitment of the intracellular components required for signal transduction *(49)*. It would seem that superantigens have evolved to mimic peptide antigens with respect to receptor clustering *(50)*, either through direct clustering events, or by the binding of superantigen homodimers to multiple MHC class II molecules, which would in turn promote T-cell clustering *(34)*. Superantigens that act as monomers and that possess only a single MHC class II binding site appear to rely on the interactions of the TCR V_α and MHC class II-β1, which increases the stability of the ternary complex to within the range seen for conventional antigen. A stable MHC/superantigen/TCR complex with an extended half-life would therefore facilitate receptor clustering.

3.4. Stimulation of Monocytes/Lymphocytes: Induction of mRNA and Proteins

Figure 4 shows a model for superantigen-induced shock. The massive T-cell proliferation induced by superantigens results in the release of high levels of a variety of cytokines both from macrophages and from T cells. These include interleukin-1 (IL-1) and tumor-necrosis factor-α (TNF-α) from macrophages and TNF-β, IL-2, and interferon-γ (IFN-γ) from T cells *(51)*. All these cytokines have deleterious effects on the host when present in high concentrations, including the production of hypotension through capillary leak (*see* **Fig. 4**) and are involved in the etiology of toxic shock, food poisoning, and scarlet fever in humans and animals. In vivo experiments with SEB show that most cytokine expression is transient and occurs within the first 12 h, whereas signals involved in proliferation such as DNA synthesis and IL-2 receptor expression are not apparent until over 24 h from SEB exposure *(52)*. Once cells have undergone DNA synthesis, they are then capable of re-expressing cytokines prior to a second round of proliferation *(53)*.

4. Roles of Superantigens in Disease

4.1. Toxic Shock Syndrome

Toxic shock syndrome (TSS) is a serious, life threatening disease resulting from an infection of a susceptible host by Staphylococci- or Streptococci-expressing superantigens in vivo. TSST-1 is the key virulence factor responsible for TSS, inducing most TSS symptoms in animals. TSST-1 is responsible for nearly all menstrual TSS cases

                                                                      Baker and Acharya

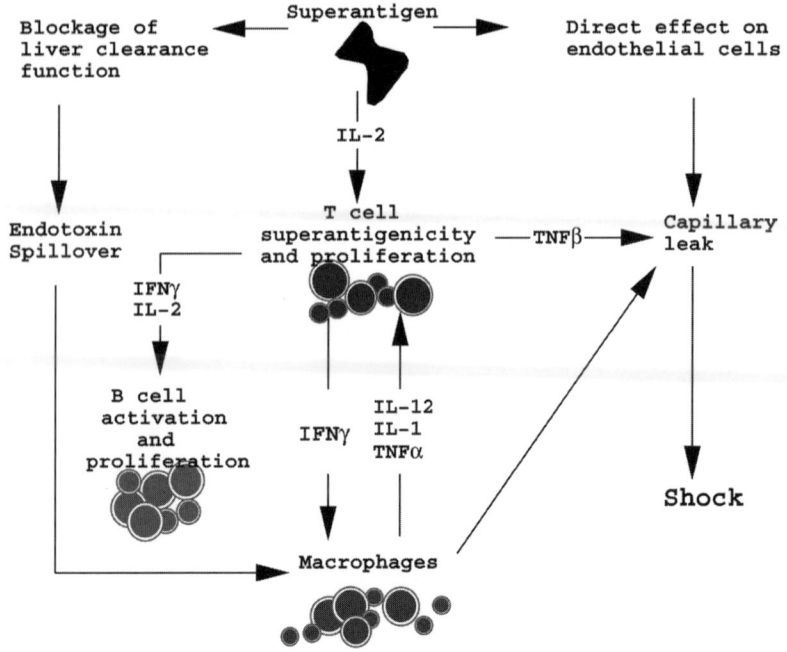

Fig. 4. The consequences of superantigen exposure. The culminative effects of superantigen on the immune system leads to hypertension and systemic shock as a result of capillary leak. Prolonged exposure to superantigen can lead to immunosuppression and tolerance.

and approx 60% of nonmenstrual Staphylococcal TSS. The remainder of the cases can be attributed primarily to SEB production, and to a lesser extent SEC and SEA *(54)*. Streptococcal TSS can be attributed mainly to SPEA *(55)*.

The pathogenesis of the disease is yet to be fully elucidated, although it is clear that toxic shock is in part a result of the superantigenic nature of the toxins. The high levels of cytokines released due to massive T-cell proliferation affect the cardiovascular system by causing extensive epithelial damage, capillary leak, and decrease in peripheral vascular resistance resulting in shock as well as reducing kidney and liver function. TSST-1 is unique among the superantigens as it is capable of crossing the epithelial barriers and subsequently inducing toxicity *(56)*. This activity is thought to be due to the unique structural features of TSST-1 that are not present in the other members of the superantigen family. The mechanism by which TSST-1 crosses the epithelial barrier could include either passive diffusion, or more likely, the use of cellular receptors *(56)*. The most pronounced structural differences between TSST-1 and the other superantigens are the lack of an α-helix in the C-terminal domain, the long N-terminal extension, and the disulphide loop. TSST-1 also has unique patches of hydrophobic and neutral residues on the front and rear of the β-barrel at the N-terminal domain. Many of these features could combine to produce a receptor specific binding site in order for TSST-1 to traverse epithelial cells and allow systemic shock.

4.2. Superantigens and Food Poisoning

Staphylococcal food poisoning (SFP) is the leading cause of microbial food-borne illness worldwide. Food sources that are contaminated most often include foods that are high in protein, salt, and sugar. Abdominal pain, nausea, vomiting, and diarrhea are commonly seen within 2–6 h of ingestion of contaminated food; the absence of fever suggests that toxemia is at most, minimal. Little is known about how superantigen structure relates with emetic and diarrhea activity. It has been suggested that the symptoms of food poisoning are a result of the high levels of cytokines released following superantigen-induced T-cell proliferation. Indeed, cancer patients receiving IL-2 therapy often experience side effects that mimic SFP. More recent work indicates that the emetic properties of these toxins are not completely correlated with their superantigenicity *(57)*. Work by Hoffman et al. *(58)* indicated that the carboxy-terminal histidine at position 225 of SEA was important for both the superantigenic and emetic activity, yet histidine 61 appears to be important only for emetic activity. Harris et al. *(57)* have identified further areas in the N-terminal region of SEA that are important for both emetic and superantigenic function. A different study on the carboxymethylation of His residues in SEB abrogates emetic activity but still induces peripheral blood cell proliferation in monkeys *(59)*, consistent with the hypothesis that the two activities are separable in staphylococcal enterotoxins. This is supported by investigations using peptides encompassing distinct regions of SEC1. Intravenous administration of one such peptide, a 22 kDa C-terminal fragment, was found to induce diarrhea but not emesis in primates *(60)*. One of the main regions of these toxins thought to be responsible for emesis is the disulphide bond and loop *(9)*. They reported that the disulphide bond itself is not an absolute requirement for emetic activity. However, conformation within or adjacent to the loop is important for emesis. Thus, it is evident that further work is required in order to assess the contribution of certain amino acids to the various biological activities shown by superantigens in the context of the diseases they cause.

4.3. Superantigens and Autoimmunity

Owing to their mode of action, superantigens have been identified as a possible candidate for one of the causative agents of autoimmune disease *(2,61)*. Because autoreactive T and B cells can easily be isolated from the peripheral blood of healthy individuals *(62,63)*, superantigens could stimulate auto-reactive T cells both locally and systemically, since they do not discriminate between autoimmune and normal lymphocytes *(64)*. Thus the delicate balance of tolerance could be broken. Although superantigens are yet to be directly implicated in human autoimmune disease, there is growing evidence to suggest their involvement. For example, SED and SED-reactive T cell lines have been shown to stimulate auto-antibody production by B cells in vitro *(65)*. It has been shown that *Staphylococcus aureus* strain AB-1 is responsible for the spontaneous outbreak of staphylococcal arthritis in a colony of rats *(66)*. When this strain was isolated from a swollen joint and injected intravenously into healthy rats, erosive, persistent arthritis developed in a majority of the rats. The arthritic lesions were characterized by the infiltration of T cells into the synovium. These T cells were later shown to be activated by a superantigen present in the infectious pathogen *(67)*.

In the absence of infection, injection of low doses of SEA or SEB induces relapsing paralysis in Experimental Autoimmune Encephalomyelitis (EAE), the animal model of multiple sclerosis *(68)*. Further studies have shown that SEB can induce MBP-specific T cells expressing different V_β to respond to myelin-antigens and mediate this relapsing paralysis *(69)*. Autoimmune conditions such as arthritis, diabetes, and multiple sclerosis are characterized by heterogeneous T cell infiltrates during active bouts of the disease. This implies that a broad spectrum of superantigens could cause this exacerbation *(70)*. Type I diabetes is associated with a retroviral superantigen, which is thought to activate and expand T cells carrying the TCR $V_\beta 7$ element, which in turn has been implicated in the pathogenesis of insulin dependent diabetes mellitus *(71)*.

Recently, the first case of type I diabetes associated with a bacterial superantigen-mediated disease was reported *(72)*. However, it still remains unclear whether superantigens are the initial trigger of autoimmune disease; as environmental factors that can change a controllable illness into one that becomes relentless for susceptible individuals.

4.4. In Vivo Models

The mouse model for toxic shock first requires the administration of D-galactosamine to sensitize the mice 2 h prior to injection of superantigen *(73,74)*. D-galactosamine destroys liver function and without its prior administration milligram quantities of toxin can be given to mice without inducing hypotension or shock. The model, therefore, is not ideal, though it provides a starting point for experiments that can be expanded with other animal models. A rabbit model with most of the symptoms characteristic of human toxic shock syndrome (TSS) excluding rash and desquamatiom can be induced by injection of TSST-1 and endotoxin *(75)*. Rabbits are first given a sublethal dose of TSST-1; it is important to pre-condition the animals because TSST-1 is lethal to unconditioned animals. Four hours after the initial dose, endotoxin is administered and the disease monitored by following the onset of TSST-1 induced fever by rectal thermometers and checking for signs of diarrhea, hypothermia, and awkward breathing. High doses of exotoxin can cause death within 3 h. It is important to note that the symptoms observed in this model are not typical of endotoxin shock, but rather, are greatly accelerated in timescale *(76)*. A variation on this rabbit model was devised using a subcutaneous infusion pump to deliver a constant toxin dose at 150 µg over 7 d period *(77)*. The highly reproducible nature of this model makes it ideal for studying the pathogenesis of TSS.

The monkey feeding test for Staphylococcal enterotoxins allows the potency of a particular sample to induce emesis and other symptoms of superantigen induced food poisoning to be assessed *(78)*. This model has been used both to test drugs designed to inhibit emesis and to determine the efficacy of vaccines designed to prevent illness in humans *(79)*.

4.5. In Vitro Models

TSST-1 pre-treated rat renal tubular epithelial cells (RTC) are sensitive to endotoxin induced necrosis at concentrations of less than 1 ng/mL *(80)*. Briefly, RTC are incubated with nontoxic levels of TSST-1 for 20 min, washed, and then exposed to endotoxin. Cytotoxicity is assessed by either trypan blue staining or by using chemiluminescence to detect reactive oxygen species (ROS) generated by those cells destroyed by endotoxin.

Direct assessment of complex formation, T-cell stimulation, and cytokine production can be assessed by using a T-cell stimulation assay. Superantigen is incubated with APCs and T-cells *(42)* and stimulation can be assessed by either incorporation of [^{3}H] thymidine into DNA and counting on a scintillation counter, which measures secreted cytokine levels, or by fluorescence-activated cell sorting (FACS). Peripheral blood mononuclear cells (PBMC) assays measure the superantigen-induced proliferation directly without the need for APCs to be present *(81)* and stimulation can be assessed as with T-cell assays.

TCR V_β analysis can be performed using the reverse dot-blot procedure *(44)*. Total TCR V_β mRNA enrichment in human peripheral blood T-cell cultures can be determined by a novel single-tube amplification technique using a redundant V_β-specific primer. Peripheral blood lymphocytes (PBL) are incubated with toxin for 3 d. TCR V_β-chain mRNA is then reverse-transcribed using a set of primers specific for the conserved region in all V_β-chain genes. A radio-labeled V_β probe is then reverse blotted onto filters containing the individual V_β-chain genes. Relative changes in V_β-chain mRNA levels from superantigen-stimulated PBL are then compared to mRNA levels in unactivated PBL.

4.6. Superantigens: Vaccines and Therapeutic Potential

Historical evidence suggested that treatment with superantigens might be of potential therapeutic value for cancer patients. Over 100 yrs ago William B. Coley administered heat-killed bacterial cultures to cancer patients *(82)*. Many of the patients who had been injected with bacteria experienced a dramatic regression in their tumors and several experienced apparent cure. It is likely that these effects can be attributed to the immunostimulatory properties of superantigens in the injected bacterial preparation. Further evidence for the involvement of supeantigens in these early experiments was provided by the attempted immunoadsorption of tumor-blocking antibodies by passing the patients' plasma over a protein A column. It was observed at the time that treatment with this preparation was accompanied by all the symptoms of superantigen-induced shock in the patient. It was later discovered that the columns were heavily contaminated with SEA and/or SEB. Protein A effectively binds several subclasses of immunoglobulins, but in contrast to SEs it has no immunoactivating properties compatible with the side effects observed in the patients. When protein A was produced recombinantly in *E. coli*, no toxic or therapeutic effects were observed. This suggestion of a therapeutic window where tolerable systemic immune activation can result in tumor regression has lead to recent attempts to specifically target superantigens towards tumors. The production of fusion proteins from tumor-specific MAbs linked to superantigens represent the modern equivalent of these historic examples.

A majority of the recent work in this field has focused on the use of SEA fused to a tumor-reactive monoclonal antibody (MAb) (83). The therapy works by targeting the superantigen directly towards the tumor; inducing infiltrating lymphocytes, the local release of tumor-suppressive cytokines, and the induction of apoptosis in tumor cells (84–86). A limitation to this approach is the accumulation of Fab-SEA fusion proteins in normal healthy tissues expressing MHC class II molecule. This causes immune activation and dose limiting toxicity (83,87).

Mutation of residues in the high-affinity MHC class II binding site reduces the systemic toxicity of the fusion protein while retaining potent anti-tumor activity (83). Similarly, several cell-based vaccines for the stimulation of immunity to metastasic cancers also employ superantigens in order to boost the immune response towards the tumour (88). Third-generation vaccines consisting of tumor cells transfected with MHC class II, CD80, and SEB genes are very effective agents for the treatment of mice with established metastasic disease.

The available data for the superantigens highlights their involvement in many diseases through one common mechanism. The production of a vaccine against bacterial superantigens could therefore lead to the abolition of such diseases. At present especially with the number of reported cases of multi-resistant Staphylococcus aureus (MRSA) on the rise, the need for a broad-spectrum vaccine or prophylactic effective against all structurally related bacterial superantigens is of paramount importance. Studies with SEA show that the MHC class II binding regions of superantigens represent the best target for site directed mutagenesis in order to produce a vaccine (89). In contrast, the TCR-binding mechanisms of superantigens are not conserved (90) and mutating a key amino acid residue in these sites may cause the acquisition of a new TCR V_β profile (41). Because MHC class II-binding residues are conserved reasonably well among the superantigens, this seems like a more sensible area to start in order to produce an effective vaccine *(89,90)*. Ulrich et al. *(90)* developed several vaccines based on conserved regions of SEA and SEB. These regions included residues in the hydrophobic pocket (Tyr89-Ala, Thr115-Ala, Glu67-Gln) and residues in the hydrophobic binding loop (Gln43-Pro, Phe44-Pro, Leu45-Arg). Immunization with these vaccines was found to protect mice and rhesus monkeys from lethal toxic shock. The antibodies produced against these vaccines also recognized and neutralized distantly related superantigens *(90)*. Other strategies for attenuating superantigen action include low molecular-weight peptides that can interfere with the binding of superantigen *via* the peptide-binding groove.

Recently, Arad et al. *(91)* reported the identification of a dodecapeptide that prevents superantigen-induced TSS in a mouse model. The peptide consisted of a highly conserved 12 residue stretch spanning residues 150–161 of SEB (β7-strand-β8-strand -α-4-helix). The peptide represents a region of no known function and is located outside of the known binding domains for both MHC class II molecules and TCR. Protected mice that survive subsequent lethal challenge with both staphylococcal and streptococcal superantigens rapidly develop protective antibodies against serologically distinct superantigens. The peptide was also shown to be effective at rescuing mice undergoing toxic shock. Similar work by Visvanathan et al. *(92)* using a peptide encompassing the same conserved region of superantigen structure plus a further 13 residues (residues 150–174) gave further insight into how these peptide work. This peptide was able to protect against lethal shock in a rabbit model and block up to 90% of superantigen-induced proliferation. Binding experiments indicated that the peptide binds tightly to MHC class II molecule, preventing the association of superantigen. Antibodies raised against this peptide were also able to block the proliferative effects of superantigens. The broad specificity of these peptides makes them an ideal vaccine/therapy for superantigen-mediated diseases. However a clear mechanism on how these peptide/s function is yet to be elucidated.

Another approach towards the inhibition of T-cell response by superantigens is the use of bispecific receptor mimics. The strategy for the design of such molecules is to incorporate structural elements of the receptors required for binding of the toxin and not as a host of the natural ligand. As a result, only toxin binding is inhibited, while the presentation of peptide antigen allowing a normal immune response is free to occur. Lehnert et al. *(93)* recently reported such a molecule from regions of DRα and TCR V_β joined together by a linker peptide that allows the two halves of the molecule to be held in correct orientations for binding of SEB. The receptor mimic inhibited SEB binding, blocked IL-2 release, and stopped T-cell proliferation. The dissociation constants for SEB binding to MHC class II-TCR complex and SEB-receptor mimic were very similar *(94)* indicating that the amount required for competitive inhibition would also be in the nanomolar range. By extending this strategy, production of bispecific receptor mimics against other superantigens should be relatively straightforward and appears to have considerable promise.

Acknowledgments

We thank our colleagues in the Structural Biology Group, Dr. Carleen M. Collins, and Dr. Laurence I. Irons for the constructive criticisms of this review. The superantigen research in K. Ravi Acharya's laboratory was supported by a Programme Grant (9540039) and Matthew D. Baker was supported by a Collaborative Post-graduate Studentship (G78/6152) from the Medical Research Council (UK).

References

1. Marrack, P. and Kappler, J. (1990) The staphylococcal enterotoxins and their relatives. *Science* **248,** 705–711.
2. Kotzin, B. L., Leung, D. Y., Kappler, J., and Marrack, P. (1993) Superantigens and their potential role in human disease. *Adv. Immunol.* **54,** 99–166.

3. White, J., Herman, A., Pullen, A. M., Kubo, R., Kappler, J. W., and Marrack, P. (1989) The V_β-specific superantigen staphylococcal enterotoxin B: stimulation of mature T cells and clonal deletion in neonatal mice. *Cell* **56,** 27–35.

4. Papageorgiou, A. C. and Acharya, K. R. (2000) Microbial superantigens: from structure to function. *Trends Microbiol.* **8,** 369–375.

5. Papageorgiou, A. C. and Acharya, K. R. (1997) Superantigens as immunomodulators: recent structural insights. *Structure* **5,** 991–996.

6. Cole, B. C., Knudtson, K. L., Oliphant, A., Sawitzke, A. D., Pole, A., Manohar, M., et al. (1996) The sequence of the Mycoplasma arthritidis superantigen, MAM: identification of functional domains and comparison with microbial superantigens and plant lectin mitogens. *J. Exp. Med.* **183,** 1105–1110.

7. Huber, B. T., Hsu, P. N., and Sutkowski, N. (1996) Virus-encoded superantigens. *Microbiol. Rev.* **60,** 473–482.

8. Huber, B. T. (1995) The role of superantigens in virus infection. *J. Clin. Immunol.* **15,** 22S–25S.

9. Hovde, C. J., Marr, J. C., Hoffmann, M. L., Hackett, S. P., Chi, Y. I., Crum, K. K., et al. (1994) Investigation of the role of the disulphide bond in the activity and structure of staphylococcal enterotoxin C1. *Mol. Microbiol.* **13,** 897–909.

10. Kline, J. B. and Collins, C. M. (1997) Analysis of the interaction between the bacterial superantigen streptococcal pyrogenic exotoxin A (SpeA) and the human T-cell receptor. *Mol. Microbiol.* **24,** 191–202.

11. Avena, R. M. and Bergdoll, M. S. (1967) Purification and some physicochemical properties of enterotoxin C, Staphylococcus aureus strain 361. *Biochemistry* **6,** 1474–1480.

12. Chu, F. S., Thadhani, K., Schantz, E. J., and Bergdoll, M. S. (1966) Purification and characterization of staphylococcal enterotoxin A. *Biochemistry* **5,** 3281–3289.

13. Ende, I. A., Terplan, G., Kickhofen, B., and Hammer, D. K. (1983) Chromatofocusing: a new method for purification of staphylococcal enterotoxins B and C1. *Appl. Environ. Microbiol.* **46,** 1323–1330.

14. Reynolds, D., Tranter, H. S., Sage, R., and Hambleton, P. (1988) Novel method for purification of staphylococcal enterotoxin A. *Appl. Environ. Microbiol.* **54,** 1761–1765.

15. Robern, H., Stavric, S., and Dickie, N. (1975) The application of QAE-Sephadex for the purification of two staphylococcal entero-

toxins. I. Purification of enterotoxin C2. *Biochim. Biophys. Acta* **393,** 148–158.

16. Brehm, R. D., Tranter, H. S., Hambleton, P., and Melling, J. (1990) Large-scale purification of staphylococcal enterotoxins A, B, and C2 by dye ligand affinity chromatography. *Appl. Environ. Microbiol.* **56,** 1067–1072.

17. Proft, T., Moffatt, S. L., Berkahn, C. J., and Fraser, J. D. (1999) Identification and characterization of novel superantigens from Streptococcus pyogenes. *J. Exp. Med.* **189,** 89–102.

18. Sundberg, E. and Jardetzky, T. S. (1999) Structural basis for HLA-DQ binding by the streptococcal superantigen SSA. *Nat. Struct. Biol.* **6,** 123–129.

19. Munson, S. H., Tremaine, M. T., Betley, M. J., and Welch, R. A. (1998) Identification and characterization of staphylococcal enterotoxin types G and I from Staphylococcus aureus. *Infect. Immun.* **66,** 3337–3348.

20. Fagin, U., Hahn, U., Grotzinger, J., Fleischer, B., Gerlach, D., Buck, F., et al. (1997) Exclusion of bioactive contaminations in Streptococcus pyogenes erythrogenic toxin A preparations by recombinant expression in *Escherichia coli. Infect. Immun.* **65,** 4725–4733.

21. Schlievert, P. M. (1988) Immunochemical assays for toxic shock syndrome toxin-1. *Methods Enzymol.* **165,** 339–344.

22. Parsonnet, J., Hickman, R. K., Eardley, D. D., and Pier, G. B. (1985) Induction of human interleukin-1 by toxic-shock-syndrome toxin-1. *J. Infect. Dis.* **151,** 514–522.

23. Sriskandan, S., Moyes, D., Buttery, L. K., Krausz, T., Evans, T. J., Polak, J., and Cohen, J. (1996) Streptococcal pyrogenic exotoxin A release, distribution, and role in a murine model of fasciitis and multiorgan failure due to Streptococcus pyogenes. *J. Infect. Dis.* **173,** 1399–1407.

24. Sriskandan, S., Moyes, D., and Cohen, J. (1996) Detection of circulating bacterial superantigen and lymphotoxin-α in patients with streptococcal toxic-shock syndrome. *Lancet* **348,** 1315–1316.

25. Jardetzky, T. S., Brown, J. H., Gorga, J. C., Stern, L. J., Urban, R. G., Chi, Y. I., et al. (1994) Three-dimensional structure of a human class II histocompatibility molecule complexed with superantigen. *Nature* **368,** 711–718.

26. Li, Y., Li, H., Dimasi, N., McCormick, J. K., Martin, R., Schuck, P.,

et al. (2001) Crystal structure of a superantigen bound to the high-affinity, zinc-dependent site on MHC class II. *Immunity* **14**, 93–104.

27. Petersson, K., Hakansson, M., Nilsson, H., Forsberg, G., Svensson, L. A., Liljas, A., and Walse, B. (2001) Crystal structure of a superantigen bound to MHC class II displays zinc and peptide dependence. *EMBO J.* **20**, 3306–3312.

28. Papageorgiou, A. C., Acharya, K. R., Shapiro, R., Passalacqua, E. F., Brehm, R. D., and Tranter, H. S. (1995) Crystal structure of the superantigen enterotoxin C2 from Staphylococcus aureus reveals a zinc-binding site. *Structure* **3**, 769–779.

29. Papageorgiou, A. C., Collins, C. M., Gutman, D. M., Kline, J. B., O'Brien, S. M., Tranter, H. S., and Acharya, K. R. (1999) Structural basis for the recognition of superantigen streptococcal pyrogenic exotoxin A (SpeA1) by MHC class II molecules and T-cell receptors. *EMBO J.* **18**, 9–21.

30. Kim, J., Urban, R. G., Strominger, J. L., and Wiley, D. C. (1994) Toxic shock syndrome toxin-1 complexed with a class II major histocompatibility molecule HLA-DR1. *Science* **266**, 1870–1874.

31. Wen, R., Broussard, D. R., Surman, S., Hogg, T. L., Blackman, M. A., and Woodland, D. L. (1997) Carboxy-terminal residues of major histocompatibility complex class II- associated peptides control the presentation of the bacterial superantigen toxic shock syndrome toxin-1 to T cells. *Eur. J. Immunol.* **27**, 772–781.

32. Fraser, J. D., Urban, R. G., Strominger, J. L., and Robinson, H. (1992) Zinc regulates the function of two superantigens. *Proc. Natl. Acad. Sci. USA* **89**, 5507–5511.

33. Abrahmsen, L., Dohlsten, M., Segren, S., Björk, P., Jonsson, E., and Kalland, T. (1995) Characterization of two distinct MHC class II binding sites in the superantigen staphylococcal enterotoxin A. *EMBO J.* **14**, 2978–2986.

34. Tiedemann, R. E., Urban, R. J., Strominger, J. L., and Fraser, J. D. (1995) Isolation of HLA-DR1. (staphylococcal enterotoxin A)2 trimers in solution. *Proc. Natl. Acad. Sci. USA* **92**, 12,156–12,159.

35. Sundstrom, M., Abrahmsen, L., Antonsson, P., Mehindate, K., Mourad, W., and Dohlsten, M. (1996) The crystal structure of staphylococcal enterotoxin type D reveals Zn^{2+}-mediated homo-dimerization. *EMBO J.* **15**, 6832–6840.

36. Roussel, A., Anderson, B. F., Baker, H. M., Fraser, J. D., and Baker, E. N. (1997) Crystal structure of the streptococcal superantigen SPE-

C: dimerization and zinc binding suggest a novel mode of interaction with MHC class II molecules. *Nat. Struct. Biol.* **4,** 635–643.

37. Hakansson, M., Petersson, K., Nilsson, H., Forsberg, G., Björk, P., Antonsson, P., and Svensson, L. A. (2000) The crystal structure of staphylococcal enterotoxin H: implications for binding properties to MHC class II and TCR molecules. *J. Mol. Biol.* **302,** 527–537.

38. Li, H., Llera, A., and Mariuzza, R. A. (1998) Structure-function studies of T-cell receptor-superantigen interactions. *Immunol Rev* **163,** 177–186.

39. Swaminathan, S., Furey, W., Pletcher, J., and Sax, M. (1992) Crystal structure of staphylococcal enterotoxin B, a superantigen. *Nature* **359,** 801–806.

40. Fields, B. A., Malchiodi, E. L., Li, H., Ysern, X., Stauffacher, C. V., Schlievert, P. M., et al. (1996) Crystal structure of a T-cell receptor β-chain complexed with a superantigen. *Nature* **384,** 188–192.

41. Kappler, J. W., Herman, A., Clements, J., and Marrack, P. (1992) Mutations defining functional regions of the superantigen staphylococcal enterotoxin B. *J. Exp. Med.* **175,** 387–396.

42. Leder, L., Llera, A., Lavoie, P. M., Lebedeva, M. I., Li, H., Sekaly, R. P., et al. (1998) A mutational analysis of the binding of staphylococcal enterotoxins B and C3 to the T cell receptor β chain and major histocompatibility complex class II. *J. Exp. Med.* **187,** 823–833.

43. Deringer, J. R., Ely, R. J., Stauffacher, C. V., and Bohach, G. A. (1996) Subtype-specific interactions of type C staphylococcal enterotoxins with the T-cell receptor. *Mol. Microbiol.* **22,** 523–534.

44. Hudson, K. R., Robinson, H., and Fraser, J. D. (1993) Two adjacent residues in staphylococcal enterotoxins A and E determine T cell receptor V_β specificity. *J. Exp. Med.* **177,** 175–184.

45. Acharya, K. R., Passalacqua, E. F., Jones, E. Y., Harlos, K., Stuart, D. I., Brehm, R. D., and Tranter, H. S. (1994) Structural basis of superantigen action inferred from crystal structure of toxic-shock syndrome toxin-1. *Nature* **367,** 94–97.

46. Deresiewicz, R. L., Woo, J., Chan, M., Finberg, R. W., and Kasper, D. L. (1994) Mutations affecting the activity of toxic shock syndrome toxin-1. *Biochemistry* **33,** 12,844–12,851.

47. Bavari, S., and Ulrich, R. G. (1995) Staphylococcal enterotoxin A and toxic shock syndrome toxin compete with CD4 for human major histocompatibility complex class II binding. *Infect. Immun.* **63,** 423–429.

48. Krakauer, T. (1995) Differential inhibitory effects of interleukin-10,

interleukin-4, and dexamethasone on staphylococcal enterotoxin-induced cytokine production and T cell activation. *J. Leukoc. Biol.* **57**, 450–454.

49. Germain, R. N. (1997) T-cell signaling: the importance of receptor clustering. *Curr. Biol.* **7**, 640–644.

50. Woodland, D. L., Wen, R., and Blackman, M. A. (1997) Why do superantigens care about peptides? *Immunol. Today* **18**, 18–22.

51. Herman, A., Kappler, J. W., Marrack, P., and Pullen, A. M. (1991) Superantigens: mechanism of T-cell stimulation and role in immune responses. *Annu. Rev. Immunol.* **9**, 745–772.

52. Picker, L. J., Singh, M. K., Zdraveski, Z., Treer, J. R., Waldrop, S. L., Bergstresser, P. R., and Maino, V. C. (1995) Direct demonstration of cytokine synthesis heterogeneity among human memory/effector T cells by flow cytometry. *Blood* **86**, 1408–1419.

53. Mehta, B. A. and Maino, V. C. (1997) Simultaneous detection of DNA synthesis and cytokine production in staphylococcal enterotoxin B activated CD4+ T lymphocytes by flow cytometry. *J. Immunol. Methods* **208**, 49–59.

54. Bernal, A., Proft, T., Fraser, J. D., and Posnett, D. N. (1999) Superantigens in human disease. *J. Clin. Immunol.* **19**, 149–157.

55. Hauser, A. R., Stevens, D. L., and Schlievert, P. M. (1991) Molecular analysis of pyrogenic exotoxins from *Streptococcus pyogenes* islates associated with toxic shock-like syndrome. *J. Clin. Microbiol.* **29**, 1562–1567.

56. Schlievert, P. M., Jablonski, L. M., Roggiani, M., Sadler, I., Callantine, S., Mitchell, D. T., et al. (2000) Pyrogenic toxin superantigen site specificity in toxic shock syndrome and food poisoning in animals. *Infect. Immun.* **68**, 3630–3634.

57. Harris, T. O. and Betley, M. J. (1995) Biological activities of staphylococcal enterotoxin type A mutants with N-terminal substitutions. *Infect. Immun.* **63**, 2133–2140.

58. Hoffman, M., Tremaine, M., Mansfield, J., and Betley, M. (1996) Biochemical and mutational analysis of the histidine residues of staphylococcal enterotoxin A. *Infect. Immun.* **64**, 885–890.

59. Alber, G., Hammer, D. K., and Fleischer, B. (1990) Relationship between enterotoxic- and T lymphocyte-stimulating activity of staphylococcal enterotoxin B. *J. Immunol.* **144**, 4501–4506.

60. Spero, L. and Morlock, B. A. (1978) Biological activities of the peptides of Staphylococcal enterotoxin C formed by limited tryptic hydrolysis. *J. Biol. Chem.* **253**, 8787–8791.

61. Friedman, S. M., Tumang, J. R., and Crow, M. K. (1993) Microbial

28   Baker and Acharya

superantigens as etiopathogenic agents in autoimmunity. *Rheum. Dis. Clin. North Am.* **19,** 207–222.

62. Hohlfeld, R., Toyka, K. V., Heininger, K., Grosse-Wilde, H., and Kalies, I. (1984) Autoimmune human T lymphocytes specific for acetylcholine receptor. *Nature* **310,** 244–246.

63. Wucherpfennig, K. W., Weiner, H. L., and Hafler, D. A. (1991) T-cell recognition of myelin basic protein. *Immunol. Today* **12,** 277–282.

64. Brocke, S., Hausmann, S., Steinman, L., and Wucherpfennig, K. W. (1998) Microbial peptides and superantigens in the pathogenesis of autoimmune diseases of the central nervous system. *Semin. Immunol.* **10,** 57–67.

65. Renno, T. and Acha-Orbea, H. (1996) Superantigens in autoimmune diseases: still more shades of gray. *Immunol Rev* **154,** 175–191.

66. Bremell, T., Lange, S., Holmdahl, R., Ryden, C., Hansson, G. K., and Tarkowski, A. (1994) Immunopathological features of rat *Staphylococcus aureus* arthritis. *Infect. Immun.* **62,** 2334–2344.

67. Bremell, T. and Tarkowski, A. (1995) Preferential induction of septic arthritis and mortality by superantigen-producing staphylococci. *Infect. Immun.* **63,** 4185–4187.

68. Brocke, S., Gaur, A., Piercy, C., Gautam, A., Gijbels, K., Fathman, C. G., and Steinman, L. (1993) Induction of relapsing paralysis in experimental autoimmune encephalomyelitis by bacterial superantigen. *Nature* **365,** 642–644.

69. Gaur, A., Fathman, C. G., Steinman, L., and Brocke, S. (1993) SEB induced anergy: modulation of immune response to T cell determinants of myoglobin and myelin basic protein. *J. Immunol.* **150,** 3062–3069.

70. Soos, J. M., Schiffenbauer, J., Torres, B. A., and Johnson, H. M. (1997) Superantigens as virulence factors in autoimmunity and immunodeficiency diseases. *Med. Hypotheses* **48,** 253–259.

71. Conrad, B., Weissmahr, R. N., Boni, J., Arcari, R., Schupbach, J., and Mach, B. (1997) A human endogenous retroviral superantigen as candidate autoimmune gene in type I diabetes. *Cell* **90,** 303–313.

72. Couper, J. J., Kallincos, N., Pollard, A., Honeyman, M., Prager, P., Harrison, L. C., and Rischmueller, M. (2000) Toxic shock syndrome associated with newly diagnosed type I diabetes. *J. Paediatr. Child Health* **36,** 279–282.

73. Miethke, T., Wahl, C., Holzmann, B., Heeg, K., and Wagner, H. (1993) Bacterial superantigens induce rapid and T cell receptor V_β-

selective down-regulation of L-selectin (gp90Mel-14) in vivo. *J. Immunol.* **151,** 6777–6782.

74. Miethke, T., Wahl, C., Regele, D., Gaus, H., Heeg, K., and Wagner, H. (1993) Superantigen mediated shock: a cytokine release syndrome. *Immunobiology* **189,** 270–284.

75. Schlievert, P. M. (1982) Enhancement of host susceptibility to lethal endotoxin shock by staphylococcal pyrogenic exotoxin type C. *Infect. Immun.* 36, 123–128.

76. Bohach, G. A. and Schlievert, P. M. (1988) Detection of endotoxin by enhancement with toxic shock syndrome toxin-1 (TSST-1). *Methods Enzymol.* **165,** 302–306.

77. Parsonnet, J., Gillis, Z. A., Richter, A. G., and Pier, G. B. (1987) A rabbit model of toxic shock syndrome that uses a constant, subcutaneous infusion of toxic shock syndrome toxin 1. *Infect. Immun.* **55,** 1070–1076.

78. Bergdoll, M. S. (1988) Monkey feeding test for staphylococcal enterotoxin. *Methods Enzymol.* **165,** 324–333.

79. Bergdoll, M. S. (1966) Immunization of Rhesus monkeys with enterotoxoid B. *J. Infect. Dis.* **116,** 191–196.

80. Keane, W. F., Gekker, G., Schlievert, P. M., and Peterson, P. K. (1986) Enhancement of endotoxin-induced isolated renal tubular cell injury by toxic shock syndrome toxin 1. *Am. J. Pathol.* **122,** 169–176.

81. Braun, M. A., Gerlach, D., Hartwig, U. F., Ozegowski, J. H., Romagne, F., Carrel, S., et al. (1993) Stimulation of human T cells by streptococcal "superantigen" erythrogenic toxins (scarlet fever toxins). *J. Immunol.* **150,** 2457–2466.

82. Kalland, T., Dohlsten, M., Lando, P., et al. (1995) In: *Bacterial Superantigens: Structure, Function and Therapeutic Potential* (Thibodeau, J. and Sekaly, R.S., eds.). Springer-Verlag, Germany, pp. 234–235.

83. Hansson, J., Ohlsson, L., Persson, R., Andersson, G., Ilback, N. G., Litton, M. J., et al. (1997) Genetically engineered superantigens as tolerable antitumor agents. *Proc. Natl. Acad. Sci. USA* **94,** 2489–2494.

84. Litton, M. J., Dohlsten, M., Lando, P. A., Kalland, T., Ohlsson, L., Andersson, J., and Andersson, U. (1996) Antibody-targeted superantigen therapy induces tumor-infiltrating lymphocytes, excessive cytokine production, and apoptosis in human colon carcinoma. *Eur. J. Immunol.* **26,** 1–9.

85. Dohlsten, M., Lando, P. A., Bjork, P., Abrahmsen, L., Ohlsson, L., Lind, P., and Kalland, T. (1995) Immunotherapy of human colon cancer by antibody-targeted superantigens. *Cancer Immunol. Immunother.* **41**, 162–168.

86. Dohlsten, M., Hansson, J., Ohlsson, L., Litton, M., and Kalland, T. (1995) Antibody-targeted superantigens are potent inducers of tumor- infiltrating T lymphocytes in vivo. *Proc. Natl. Acad. Sci. USA* **92**, 9791–9795.

87. Dohlsten, M., Kalland, T., Gunnarsson, P., Antonsson, P., Molander, A., Olsson, J., et al. (1998) Man-made superantigens: Tumor-selective agents for T-cell-based therapy. *Adv. Drug Deliv. Rev.* **31**, 131–142.

88. Ostrand-Rosenberg, S., Pulaski, B. A., Clements, V. K., Qi, L., Pipeling, M. R., and Hanyok, L. A. (1999) Cell-based vaccines for the stimulation of immunity to metastatic cancers. *Immunol. Rev.* **170**, 101–114.

89. Bavari, S., Dyas, B., and Ulrich, R. G. (1996) Superantigen vaccines: a comparative study of genetically attenuated receptor-binding mutants of staphylococcal enterotoxin A. *J. Infect. Dis.* **174**, 338–345.

90. Ulrich, R. G., Olson, M. A., and Bavari, S. (1998) Development of engineered vaccines effective against structurally related bacterial superantigens. *Vaccine* **16**, 1857–1864.

91. Arad, G., Levy, R., Hillman, D., and Kaempfer, R. (2000) Superantigen antagonist protects against lethal shock and defines a new domain for T-cell activation [see comments]. *Nat. Med.* **6**, 414–421.

92. Visvanathan, K., Charles, A., Bannan, J., Pugach, P., Kashfi, K., and Zabriskie, J. B. (2001) Inhibition of bacterial superantigens by peptides and antibodies. *Infect. Immun.* **69**, 875–884.

93. Lehnert, N. M., Allen, D. L., Allen, B. L., Catasti, P., Shiflett, P. R., Chen, M., et al. (2001) Structure-based design of a bispecific receptor mimic that inhibits T cell responses to a superantigen. *Biochemistry* **40**, 4222–4228.

94. Redpath, S., Alam, S. M., Lin, C. M., O'Rourke, A. M., and Gascoigne, N. R. (1999) Cutting edge: trimolecular interaction of TCR with MHC class II and bacterial superantigen shows a similar affinity to MHC:peptide ligands. *J. Immunol.* **163**, 6–10.

95. Sundstrom, M., Hallen, D., Svensson, A., Schad, E., Dohlsten, M., and Abrahmsen, L. (1996) The Co-crystal structure of staphylococcal enterotoxin type A with Zn^{2+} at 2.7 Å resolution. Implications

for major histocompatibility complex class II binding. *J. Biol. Chem.* **271,** 32,212–32,216.

96. Papageorgiou, A. C., Tranter, H. S., and Acharya, K. R. (1998) Crystal structure of microbial superantigen staphylococcal enterotoxin B at 1.5Å resolution: implications for superantigen recognition by MHC class II molecules and T-cell receptors. *J. Mol. Biol.* **277,** 61–79.

97. Papageorgiou, A. C., Brehm, R. D., Leonidas, D. D., Tranter, H. S., and Acharya, K. R. (1996) The refined crystal structure of toxic shock syndrome toxin-1 at 2.07Å resolution. *J. Mol. Biol.* **260,** 553–569.

98. Earhart, C. A., Vath, G. M., Roggiani, M., Schlievert, P. M., and Ohlendorf, D. H. (2000) Structure of streptococcal pyrogenic exotoxin A reveals a novel metal cluster. *Protein Sci.* **9,** 1847–1851.

99. Baker, M., Gutman D. M., Papageorgiou A. C., Collins C. M., and Acharya K. R. (2001) Structural features of a zinc binding site in the superantigen streptococcal pyrogenic exotoxin A1 (SpeA1): implications for MHC class II recognition. *Protein Sci.* **10,** 1268–1273.

100. Proft, T., Moffatt, S. L., Weller, K. D., Paterson, A., Martin, D., and Fraser, J. D. (2000) The streptococcal superantigen SMEZ exhibits wide allelic variation, mosaic structure, and significant antigenic variation. *J. Exp. Med.* **191,** 1765–1776.

101. Gerlach, D., Fleischer, B., Wagner, M., Schmidt, K., Vettermann, S., and Reichardt, W. (2000) Purification and biochemical characterization of a basic superantigen (SPEX/SMEZ3) from Streptococcus pyogenes. *FEMS Microbiol. Lett.* **188,** 153–163.

2

Expression, Purification, and Detection of Novel Streptococcal Superantigens

John K. McCormick and Patrick M. Schlievert

1. Introduction

Superantigens (SAgs) are a class of bacterial or viral proteins that aberrantly alter immune system function through simultaneous interaction with lateral surfaces of major histocompatibility (MHC) class II molecules on antigen presenting cells, and to particular variable regions of the T-cell antigen receptor (TCR) β-chain. Among the secreted virulence factors from group A streptococci are the streptococcal pyrogenic exotoxins (SPEs), also commonly known as erythrogenic toxins or scarlet fever toxins. Together with the enterotoxins and toxic shock syndrome toxin-1 (TSST-1) from *Staphylococcus aureus*, the SPEs belong to a larger family of related exotoxins collectively known as the "pyrogenic toxin" class of superantigens, which share functional activities, similar amino acid sequences, and conserved three-dimensional structures *(1,2)*. Due to their notable association with scarlet fever and streptococcal toxic shock syndrome (TSS), SPE A *(3,4)* and SPE C *(5)* are generally considered to be the prototypical streptococcal superantigens.

Genome sequencing projects have recently revealed that group A streptococci possess genes encoding multiple superantigen sero-

From: *Methods in Molecular Biology, vol. 214: Superantigen Protocols*
Edited by: T. Krakauer © Humana Press Inc., Totowa, NJ

types *(6)*. From an early search of the incomplete *S. pyogenes* SF370 genome, Proft and colleagues characterized two novel streptococcal superantigens, termed SPE G and SPE H, and identified a portion of the *SPE J* gene *(7)*. Both SPE I *(8)* and SPE J *(8,9)* have been characterized since then, and including the streptococcal superantigen (SSA) *(10)* and the multiple streptococcal mitogenic exotoxin Z (SMEZ) serotypes *(11,12)*, there are eight described streptococcal superantigens. For discussion purposes, SPE A and SPE C will be referred to as the prototypical streptococcal superantigens while SPE serotypes G, H, I, J, SSA, and SMEZ will be referred to as novel streptococcal superantigens. Although SPE B and SPE F share the "SPE" nomenclature, these proteins have enzymatic activity (protease and DNAse, respectively) and neither shares significant amino acid homology to the other streptococcal superantigens. Superantigen activity of both SPE B and SPE F remains debated in the literature.

The potency of bacterial superantigens borders on the absurd where significant T cell proliferation can be detected below the picogram (10^{-12} g)/mL range. Owing to this extreme potency, many debates exist in the literature regarding the ability of a novel protein to function as a superantigen that stem from the possibility that the protein in question was contaminated with trace amounts of genuine superantigen. For this reason, and the apparent ability of streptococci to produce multiple superantigens, it is prudent to obtain recombinant superantigen proteins expressed from *Escherichia coli* for characterization of biological activities. In this chapter, we will focus on two methods used in our laboratory to purify novel streptococcal superantigens for further functional, biochemical, and immunological characterization, and will also discuss various standard methods used for their detection.

2. Materials

1. Bacterial strains: We typically do our cloning in *E. coli* XL1-blue (Stratagene, Cedar Creek, TX) but other commonly used cloning strains are acceptable. We do our recombinant protein expression in

E. coli BL21 (DE3) (Novagen, Madison, WI). This strain harbors the DE3 lysogen, which encodes the T7 RNA polymerase under inducible control by isopropyl β-D-galactopyranoside (IPTG). Thus, strains that contain the gene to be expressed under control of the T7 promoter can be induced by the addition of IPTG.

2. Plasmids: For all of our streptococcal superantigen expression work, we have used the pET28 plasmid series (Novagen).

3. Media: We routinely grow *E. coli* in Luria-Bertani (LB) media *(13)* and although for protein expression we use a dialyzed beef heart medium *(14)*, growth in LB or other standard *E. coli* medium is acceptable.

4. Water: We use either double-distilled or MilliQ filtered H_2O for all solutions and procedures after growth of the bacteria.

5. Chemicals: We obtain NaCl, Tris-HCl, $NiSO_4$, imidazole, and urea from Sigma Chemical Co. (St. Louis, MO).

6. Antibiotics: For cloning and plasmid maintenance of pET28, we use kanamycin (Sigma) at 50 μg/mL. Stocks are made at 50 mg/mL in MilliQ water, filter sterilized (0.22 μm) and stored at –20°C.

7. IPTG: For induction of gene expression in *E. coli* BL21 (DE3) we use IPTG (Sigma) at 0.2 mM. Stocks are made at 200 mg/mL in MilliQ water, filter-sterilized (0.22 μm) and stored at –20°C.

8. Ethanol: We use 200 proof ethanol that does not contain other additives.

9. Dialysis tubing: We use both 6000–8000 (23 × 14.6 mm) and 12,000–14,000 (45 × 29 mm) molecular-weight cut-off dialysis tubing (Spectrum Laboratories Inc., Rancho Dominguez, CA).

10. Preparative Isoelectric focusing (IEF) apparatus: We use a LKB Multiphor 2117 electrophoresis module (Amersham Pharmacia Biotech, Piscataway, NJ). Other commercial available preparative isoelectric focussing equipment should also be acceptable (e.g., Biorad) *(15)*.

11. Sephadex: For preparative IEF, we use Sephadex G-75 (Sigma) that has been swelled in water, exhaustively washed with absolute ethanol, and dried.

12. Ampholytes: We use 3.5–10 pH gradient and 6.0–8.0 pH gradient ampholytes (Amersham Pharmacia Biotech AB, Sweden).

13. Nickel column: We use the His-Bind Resin and buffer kit (Novagen) for purification of 6× His-tagged proteins.

14. Charge buffer: 50 mM $NiSO_4$.

15. Binding buffer: 500 mM NaCl, 20 mM Tris-HCl, pH 7.9.
16. Phosphate-buffered saline (PBS): 5 mM Na$_2$HPO$_4$/NaH$_2$PO$_4$, 150 mM NaCl, pH 7.2.

3. Methods

This section describes two methods used in our laboratory to purify novel streptococcal superantigens, and discusses standard methods used for their detection. The two purification methods differ in respect to the presence or absence of an affinity tag engineered onto the N-terminus of the protein to aid in purification. Despite the methods discussed here, novel streptococcal superantigens have also been purified from culture supernatants using affinity chromatography with anti-superantigen IgG conjugated Sepharose (e.g., SSA) *(10)* or ammonium sulfate precipitation, chromatofocusing, and hydrophobic interaction (e.g., SMEZ) *(11)*. Furthermore, novel streptococcal superantigens have be expressed as glutathione-S-transferase (GST) fusion proteins in *E. coli* and purified using glutathione (GSH) agarose followed by cation exchange chromatography (e.g., SPEs G, H, I, J) *(7,8,12,16)*.

3.1. Purification of Native (Untagged) Streptococcal Superantigens

This section describes the methods we have used to purify novel streptococcal superantigens without the aid of an affinity tag. In our experience, inclusion of DNA encoding the superantigen signal peptide in the expression plasmid results in very poor yields of protein. Thus, we clone all of our genes lacking the signal peptide. Briefly, superantigen genes are cloned by polymerase chain reaction (PCR) into the pET28 plasmid. The forward primer incorporates a *Nco*I restriction site onto the PCR product while the reverse primer incorporates a *Bam*HI restriction site following the stop codon of the gene. The *Nco*I site is engineered to allow for an in frame translational fusion with the ATG start codon encoded within the restriction site (CC<u>ATG</u>G). Clones are verified by restriction digests and

DNA sequencing. Alternatively, if the gene contains an internal *Nco*I site, *Nde*I can be used with this vector. Other than this, cloning procedures are beyond the scope of this chapter. Once the proper clone is obtained and transformed into *E. coli* BL21 (DE3), proceed as follows:

1. Grow *E. coli* BL21 (DE3) containing the appropriate plasmid overnight at 37°C with shaking in 50 mL of LB broth containing 50 µg/mL kanamycin.

2. The following morning, subculture the culture at 1% into fresh prewarmed (37°C) beef heart medium or other suitable medium containing 50 µg/mL kanamycin. We typically grow 1200 mL of culture but the method can be scaled up or down as desired. A typical yield following the protocol is about 5 mg of pure superantigen per liter of culture.

3. Monitor growth until the absorbance at 600 nm is approx 0.5. Induce superantigen gene expression with the addition of IPTG (0.2 m*M*). Continue to grow 3–4 h.

4. Precipitate the cultures with 4 volumes of absolute ethanol (80% final concentration). This step causes lysis and dehydration of the *E. coli* cells releasing intracellular protein. This concentration of ethanol typically results in the differential precipitation of proteins greater than ~10,000 Da. Proteins are generally precipitated at 4°C for 2 or more days.

5. The ethanol is poured or siphoned off and the cell debris is concentrated by centrifugation.

6. Concentrated crude protein and cell debris is dried and resuspended in water; the precipitated superantigen protein will resolubilize. Culture supernatants (up to approx 10 L) are concentrated to 50 mL.

7. Centrifuge the cell debris at 10,000*g*, retain the supernatant, and dialyze (12,000–14,000 molecular weight cut off) the supernatant against 2 L of water overnight at 4°C.

8. We run two consecutive separations via flatbed isoelectric focussing (pH 3.0–10.0 ampholytes and pH 6.0–8.0 ampholytes) with a LKB Multiphor 2117 electrophoresis apparatus using Sephadex G-75. Ampholytes are added at 5% to a total sample volume of 50 –75 mL. Sephadex is added to achieve a semi-solid support, which is poured onto the IEF plates to achieve a smooth, flat layer. The IEF gradient is run overnight (≥18 h) at 1000V, 8W, and 20mA. The initial

3.5–10.0 pH gradient removes a substantial amount of cell debris and contaminants (brown color at the acidic end of the gradient).

9. The visible band (due to a change in refractive index of the focused toxin in high concentration) is harvested. If an band is not visible, the entire basic end of the IEF (except for the brown acidic end) is harvested.

10. The fraction is usually refocused in a pH 6.0–8.0 gradient under the same conditions used for the 3.5–10.0 pH gradient. Residual 3.5–10.0 pH ampholytes are not removed. For some superantigens with a lower pI (e.g., SPE A or SSA) we use pH 4.0–6.0 ampholytes for the second gradient.

11. The visible band is harvested, Sephadex is removed by filtering through a syringe containing glass wool, and ampholytes are removed by extensive dialysis against water (4 d, 4°C) with 6,000–8,000 molecular-weight cut-off dialysis tubing (*see* **Note 1**). If a visible band is not seen, the Sephadex gel will require fractionating and the various fractions can be screened by antibody or sodium dodecyl sulfate polyacrylamide gel electrophoresis (SDS-PAGE).

12. To assess purity, we run 10 µL of each sample on a 15% SDS-PAGE. **Figure 1** shows an example of this purification procedure for recombinant SPE J *(9)*.

3.2. Purification of 6× His-Tagged Streptococcal Superantigens

This procedure generally follows the His-Bind kit protocol by Novagen (www.novagen.com) with small modifications.

1. Repeat **steps 1–3** from **Subheading 3.1.**

2. Pellet the cells by centrifugation and wash once with binding buffer. Although the manufacturer's protocols suggest using 40 mM imidazole in the binding buffer, we omit imidazole from the binding buffer.

3. Resuspend the cells at 50× concentration in binding buffer.

4. Lyse the cells with 4 rounds of sonication on ice, or alternatively using a French Press.

5. Spin down cell debris and filter (0.45 µm) the supernatant. We generally do not experience inclusion body formation with the streptococcal superantigens from this procedure, but if soluble protein yields are poor, the bacterial pellet should be solubilized in 6 M urea and checked for protein of the expected size (*see* **Note 2**).

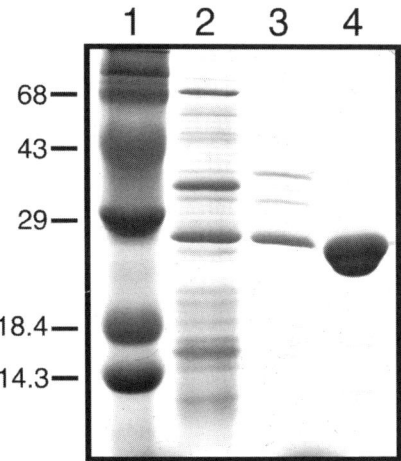

Fig. 1. Purification of streptococcal pyrogenic exotoxin J by ethanol precipitation and preparative isoelectric focusing. Shown is a 15% SDS-polyacrylamide gel stained with Coomassie brilliant blue. Lane 1, molecular-weight marker; lane 2, ethanol precipitated *E. coli* cell lysate; lane 3, protein preparation after pH 3.5–10.0 isoelectric focusing gradient; lane 4, protein preparation after pH 6.0–8.0 isoelectric focusing gradient.

6. Prepare the nickel column by gently resuspending the resin and pipeting the matrix into a standard column. The binding capacity of this column is approx 8 mg of recombinant protein per mL of resin and we generally use 1 mL of matrix for every 100 mL of *E. coli* culture. The resin can be reused for multiple purification runs of the same superantigen.

7. For 1 mL of resin we wash with 3 mL of H_2O, 5 mL of charge buffer, and 5 mL of binding buffer (*see* **Note 3**).

8. Because the loading volume for the nickel column is not an issue, dilute the sample 10× in binding buffer to dilute any remaining salts in the supernatant. Load 20 mL of diluted sample per 1 mL of column matrix. Collect the run through fraction.

9. Wash the column with 5 mL each of:
   a. Binding buffer;
   b. Binding buffer containing 30 m*M* imidazole;
   c. Binding buffer containing 60 m*M* imidazole; and
   d. Binding buffer containing 200 m*M* imidazole.
   Collect all fractions. The manufacturer's protocols recommend

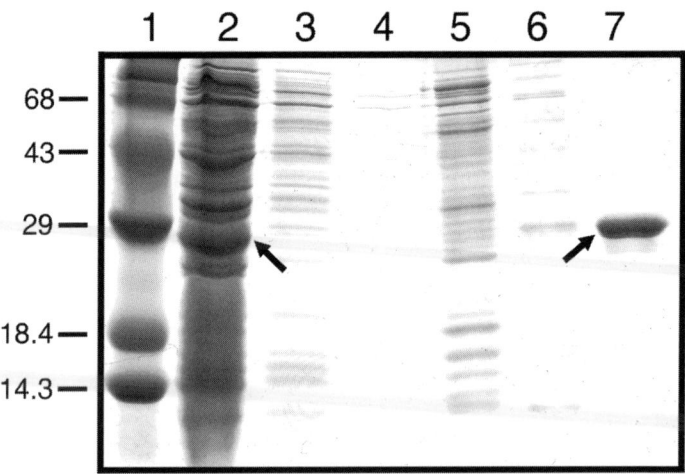

Fig. 2. Purification of 6× His-tagged streptococcal pyrogenic exotoxin G by nickel chelation chromatography. Shown is a 15% SDS-polyacrylamide gel stained with Coomassie brilliant blue. Lane 1, molecular-weight marker; lane 2, *E. coli* cell lysate; lane 3, fall through fraction after loading onto nickel column; lane 4, binding buffer wash fraction (0 mM imidazole), lane 5, 30 mM imidazole wash fraction; lane 6, 60 mM imidazaole wash fraction; lane 7, 200 mM elution fraction. Arrows indicate SPE G in the crude cell lysate and purified SPE G in the 200 mM imidazole fraction.

elution of the protein with 1 M imidazole but 200 mM is typically sufficient.

10. Run 10 µL of each sample on a 15% SDS-PAGE to assess purity. **Figure 2** shows an example of this purification procedure for recombinant 6× His-tagged SPE G. If cleavage of the 6× His-tag is desired, we suggest the Thrombin Cleavage Capture Kit (Novagen). Proteins are dialyzed against PBS before use in biological assays.

3.3. Detection of Novel Streptococcal Superantigens

We generally use a few standard techniques for the detection of the novel streptococcal superantigens during purification but these techniques can also be used for superantigen detection from clinical strains of group A streptococci. For the rapid detection of the presence of a streptococcal superantigen in high concentration

(>10 µg/mL) we use the Ouchterlony (double-immune diffusion) technique *(17)*. Gels for double immunodiffusion are prepared with 0.75% agarose in PBS. Melted agarose is poured onto glass slides (4.5 mL/slide), solidified and 4 mm diameter wells are punched 4 mm apart in a hexagonal pattern. Twenty µL of each sample is placed in the outside wells and superantigen specific antisera is added to the center well. After approx 4 h incubation at 37°C, precipitin areas are indicative of superantigen reactive with the antiserum. For the detection of small amounts of a streptococcal superantigen we use Western-blot analysis, which is a standard procedure and is beyond the scope of this chapter.

The recombinant superantigens should be of sufficient purity (*see* **Figs. 1** and **2**) to perform most experiments including biological assays and immunizations. However, our structural biology collaborators many add a final "polishing" step prior to setting up crystallization plates *(18)*.

4. Notes

1. Following purification of superantigen by preparative IEF, we remove ampholytes by dialysis. We typically do not extend the dialysis period past 4 d because in our experience the protein may precipitate as an insoluble form that we have not been able to satisfactorily solublilize.

2. During expression of recombinant protein from BL21 (DE3), occasionally the clone will no longer produce recombinant protein for reasons that are not readily clear. If this occurs, we generally retransform new BL21 (DE3) cells with the original plasmid and repeat the expression. Alternatively, if soluble protein levels of the superantigen in the crude extract are low, the pellet should be checked for inclusion body formation by solubilization in 8 *M* Urea. Because the affects of superantigen denaturation and subsequent refolding on superantigen function is unknown, we suggest growing bacteria at 30°C or using less IPTG for induction if inclusion body formation occurs.

3. It is important to avoid β-Mercaptoethanol, dithiothreitol (DTT), and EDTA in the binding buffer for use with His Bind resins because the reducing agents will precipitate the Ni^{2+} and EDTA will chelate the

Ni^{2+} from the column. Due to the extreme potency of these toxins, we do not use the same resin for different superantigen purifications.

Acknowledgments

This work was supported by USPHS grant HL36611 from NIH to Patrick M. Schlievert.

References

1. Kotb, M. (1995) Bacterial pyrogenic exotoxins as superantigens. *Clin. Microbiol. Rev.* **8,** 411–426.
2. McCormick, J. K., Yarwood, J. M., and Schlievert, P. M. (2001) Toxic shock syndrome and bacterial superantigens: an update. *Ann. Rev. Microbiol.* **55,** 77–104.
3. Weeks, C. R., and Ferretti, J. J. (1986) Nucleotide sequence of the type A streptococcal exotoxin (erythrogenic toxin) gene from Streptococcus pyogenes bacteriophage T12. *Infect. Immun.* **52,** 144–150.
4. Johnson, L. P., L'Italien, J. J., and Schlievert, P. M. (1986) Streptococcal pyrogenic exotoxin type A (scarlet fever toxin) is related to Staphylococcus aureus enterotoxin B. *Mol. Gen. Genet.* **203,** 354–356.
5. Goshorn, S. C. and Schlievert, P. M. (1988) Nucleotide sequence of streptococcal pyrogenic exotoxin type C. *Infect. Immun.* **56,** 2518–2520.
6. Ferretti, J. J., McShan, W. M., Ajdic, D., Savic, D. J., Savic, G., Lyon, K., et al. (2001) Complete genome sequence of an M1 strain of Streptococcus pyogenes. *Proc. Natl. Acad. Sci. USA* **98,** 4658–4663.
7. Proft, T., Moffatt, S. L., Berkahn, C. J., and Fraser, J. D. (1999) Identification and characterization of novel superantigens from *Streptococcus pyogenes. J. Exp. Med.* **189,** 89–102.
8. Proft, T., Arcus, V. L., Handley, V., Baker, E. N., and Fraser, J. D. (2001) Immunological and Biochemical Characterization of Streptococcal Pyrogenic Exotoxins I and J (SPE-I and SPE-J) from *Streptococcus pyogenes. J. Immunol.* **166,** 6711–6719.
9. McCormick, J. K., Pragman, A. A., Stolpa, J. C., Leung, D. Y., and Schlievert, P. M. (2001) Functional characterization of streptococcal pyrogenic exotoxin J, a novel superantigen. *Infect. Immun.* **69,** 1381–1388.

10. Mollick, J. A., Miller, G. G., Musser, J. M., Cook, R. G., Grossman, D., and Rich, R. R. (1993) A novel superantigen isolated from pathogenic strains of *Streptococcus pyogenes* with aminoterminal homology to staphylococcal enterotoxins B and C. *J. Clin. Invest.* **92,** 710–719.

11. Kamezawa, Y., Nakahara, T., Nakano, S., Abe, Y., Nozaki-Renard, J., and Isono, T. (1997) Streptococcal mitogenic exotoxin Z, a novel acidic superantigenic toxin produced by a T1 strain of Streptococcus pyogenes. *Infect. Immun.* **65,** 3828–3833.

12. Proft, T., Moffatt, S. L., Weller, K. D., Paterson, A., Martin, D., and Fraser, J. D. (2000) The streptococcal superantigen SMEZ exhibits wide allelic variation, mosaic structure, and significant antigenic variation. *J. Exp. Med.* **191,** 1765–1776.

13. Sambrook, J., Fritsch, E. F., and Maniatis, T. (1989) *Molecular Cloning: A Laboratory Manual,* 2nd ed. Cold Spring Harbor Laboratory Press, Cold Spring Harbor, NY.

14. Schlievert, P. M., Shands, K. N., Dan, B. B., Schmid, G. P., and Nishimura, R. D. (1981) Identification and characterization of an exotoxin from Staphylococcus aureus associated with toxic-shock syndrome. *J. Infect. Dis.* **143,** 509–516.

15. Kum, W. W., Laupland, K. B., See, R. H., and Chow, A. W. (1993) Improved purification and biologic activities of staphylococcal toxic shock syndrome toxin 1. *J. Clin. Microbiol.* **31,** 2654–2660.

16. Arcus, V. L., Proft, T., Sigrell, J. A., Baker, H. M., Fraser, J. D., and Baker,E. N. (2000) Conservation and variation in superantigen structure and activity highlighted by the three-dimensional structures of two new superantigens from Streptococcus pyogenes. *J. Mol. Biol.* **299,** 157–168.

17. Ouchterlony, O. (1962) Diffusion-in-gel methods for immunoogical analysis. *Prog. Allergy* **6,** 30.

18. Li, Y., Li, H., Dimasi, N., McCormick, J. K., Martin, R., Schuck, P., et al. (2001) Crystal structure of a superantigen bound to the high-affinity, zinc- dependent site on MHC class II. *Immunity* **14,** 93–104.

3

Flow Cytometric Detection of MMTV Superantigens

Gary Winslow

1. Introduction

1.1. Expression of Viral Superantigens

Mouse mammary tumor viral superantigens (vSAgs) are produced by germline-encoded proviruses and infectious viruses (for reviews *see* **refs.** *1,2*). Like other superantigens, they interact with class II major histocompatiblity complex (MHC) proteins and trigger T-cell proliferation via recognition of particular variable elements (V_β) of the T-cell receptor (TCR). Prior to the discovery of their viral origin, the provirus-encoded vSAgs were referred to as Mls (minor lymphocyte stimulatory) antigens *(3)*. Unlike the bacterial superantigens, which are produced as small soluble proteins, the vSAgs are produced as membrane glycoproteins that transit the exocytic pathway and undergo partial proteolytic processing by cellular endoproteases *(4)*. Proteolytic processing appears to be necessary for vSAgs to activate T cells *(5–7)*, and available data suggest that a soluble carboxy terminal processing product may be sufficient for vSAg function *(8)*. The vSAgs require class II MHC proteins to be presented to T cells *(9)*, although not necessarily for surface expression *(8)*.

From: *Methods in Molecular Biology, vol. 214: Superantigen Protocols*
Edited by: T. Krakauer © Humana Press Inc., Totowa, NJ

Mouse mammary tumor proviruses are carried by all common inbred laboratory mouse strains, but the particular proviruses encoded by any given strain are highly variable (for review *see* ref. *10*). In addition, several mouse strains harbor exogenous viruses that are maintained by horizontal transmission *(11)*. The vSAgs of both proviral and exogenous origins are highly conserved overall, but they exhibit significant divergence in a region of approx 30 amino acids at the immediate carboxy terminus. Subfamilies of vSAgs that are similar in this region share T-cell V_β specificity *(4)*, so this region likely defines the interaction with the T-cell receptor. vSAg-specific antibodies have therefore been generated by targeting these regions. Nomenclature of the vSAgs of proviral origin follows the designation of the provirus (e.g., vSAg7 from MMTV7) or, for exogenous retroviruses, the mouse strain that was initially found to harbor the virus (e.g., vSAg[SW]) *(12)*.

1.2. Detection of Viral Superantigens

The vSAgs are highly stimulatory for T cells, which probably explains why they are expressed on the surface of antigen-presenting cells (APCs) at low levels relative to other lymphocyte surface markers, such as class II MHC proteins. The characteristic low surface expression likely hampered early attempts to generate vSAg antibodies. vSAg antibodies had been unavailable prior to the identification of the genetic origin of the vSAgs and the elucidation of their amino acid sequences, and all of the vSAg antibodies that have been described have been generated against synthetic vSAg peptides. No antibodies have been reported to have been generated against a native superantigen.

Although evidence indicates that vSAgs are expressed on thymic and tissue dendritic cells *(13)*, and CD8 T cells *(14)*, flow cytometric detection of vSAgs on normal APCs has only been demonstrated using lipopolysaccharide (LPS) stimulated B cells *(15)*. vSAgs have been more readily detected in tumor cell lines engineered to express vSAgs under the regulation of viral promoters, but vSAg surface expression is relatively low even in these lines. Most newly synthesized vSAg is degraded in the endoplasmic reticulum *(16)* and has a short half-life *(17)*. It is possible, nevertheless, to detect surface expression of vSAgs on normal APCs, and this chapter describes a technique suitable for detecting vSAg expression on LPS stimulated B cells, and on tumor cell lines, using flow cytometry.

2. Materials

2.1. Mice and vSAg Expressing Cell Lines

1. Inbred mouse strains were obtained from commercial vendors (Jackson Laboratories, Bar Harbor, ME). It is important that appropriate strains be used for the detection of particular endogenous vSAgs (*see* **Note 1**).
2. Recombinant cell lines that express various vSAgs were generated in the author's laboratory using the vSAg7 coding sequence that was inserted into a human β-actin expression vector, or the vector pSRαpuro *(5)*. The vSAg described in this method (vSAg7, from MMTV7) was expressed in Chinese Hamster Ovary cells (CHO) that had also been engineered to express the class II protein IE^k *(5)*, which is required for vSAg stimulation of T cells. Expression of other vSAgs in tumor cells has been reported *(18,19)*.

2.2. Cell Culture

1. Complete Tumor Medium (CTM): Minimal Essential Medium (Invitrogen Life Technologies, Carlsbad, CA) and is supplemented with 10% fetal calf serum (FCS), 10 µM β-Mercaptoethanol, 10% Mishell-Dutton Nutrient cocktail *(20)*, 100 µg/mL gentamycin, 100 U/mL penicillin G, and 200 µg/mL streptomycin sulfate (Sigma Chemical, St. Louis, MO). Store reagents at 4°C and use complete media within 2 wk.
2. HBSS is from Invitrogen Life Technologies.
3. Lipopolysaccharide is (from *Salmonella typhosa*; Sigma). Stock solution is made in HBSS at 1 mg/mL and sterile filtered. Store at –20°C.
4. Erythrocyte lysis solution: 150 m*M* ammonium chloride, 0.73 m*M* potassium phosphate. Filter and store at 4°C.
5. Cell strainers (100-µm nylon) are available from Becton Dickinson Labware (Franklin Lakes, NJ).

6. Trypsin/EDTA solution is from Invitrogen Life Technologies. It is stable when stored at 4°C.
7. Antibiotic G418 sulfate is obtained from Invitrogen Life Technologies; puromycin is from Sigma.

2.3. Antibodies

1. The monoclonal vSAg7 antibody is available from the author. A vSAg1 antibody is available commercially (BD Pharmingen), although it was reported that this antibody did not detect vSAgs on LPS activated B cells *(21)*. Polyclonal rabbit vSAg antiserum has also been used to detect vSAgs on transfectant cell lines *(18)*. Monoclonal antibodies (MAbs) are typically used at 1–10 µg/mL. Stock solutions of antibodies should be stored at 4°C. Diluted working solutions should be made at 3X final concentration and stored at 4°C for less than 2 wk.
2. The MHC class II IE$^{k/d}$ antibody 14-4-4 (FITC-conjugated) is available from BD Pharmingen (San Diego, CA; *see* **Note 2**).

2.4. Flow Cytometry

1. Phycoerythrin-coupled streptavidin is from BD Pharmingen. This reagent should be titrated using a well-characterized antibody to determine optimal final dilution suitable for flow cytometric analyses. Working solutions should be made at 5× final concentration. These are typically stable for several months when stored at 4°C.
2. 96-well V-bottom plates are from Nalge Nunc International (Rochester, NY).
3. Wash buffer: phosphate buffered saline, pH 7.2, containing 2% FSC, and 0.1% sodium azide. It is stable when stored at 4°C.
4. Fc blocking solution: 100 µg/mL human gamma globulin, or normal mouse serum, and/or anti-CD16/CD32 (FcγRII/RIII specific antibody 2.4G2, available from BD Pharmingen; use at 1:500 dilution; *see* **Note 3**).

3. Methods

3.1. Induction of vSAg Expression by B Cells

1. Harvest the spleen of one mouse. Obtain splenocytes by passing the tissue through a 100-µm nylon mesh using a plunger from a syringe.

Rinse the mesh with HBSS and transfer the cells to a 15-mL conical centrifuge tube.

2. Centrifuge (1000g) and aspirate supernatant.
3. Lyse erythrocytes by resuspending the spleen cells in the erythrocyte lysis solution (0.5 mL/spleen) and incubating at 37°C for 5 min. At the end of the incubation, add 10 mL HBSS/spleen, and centrifuge at 1000g for 5 min.
4. Aspirate the supernatant and wash once with HBSS.
5. Resuspend the spleen cells in CTM and transfer to a culture flask containing CTM to a final concentration of 2×10^6 cells/mL.
6. Add LPS to 10 µg/mL (*see* **Note 4**).
7. Incubate at 37°C for 24–48 h prior to harvesting for flow cytometry.

3.2. Harvest of vSAg Expressing Transfectants

1. Culture vSAg expressing cell lines (e.g., CHIE/S7) in CTM under appropriate drug selection (for CHIE/S7 use G418 at 0.5 mg/mL and puromycin at 25 µg/mL) (*see* **Note 5**).
2. To harvest adherent cell lines, aspirate media from the flask, and add sufficient trypsin/EDTA solution to cover the bottom of the flask. Incubate at 37°C only long enough to detach adherent cells from the flask.
3. Immediately transfer the trypsinized cells to BSS containing 10% FCS, or CTM. Centrifuge at 1000g for 5 min.
4. Resuspend the cells in CTM at a concentration of $1–5 \times 10^6$/mL and incubate at 37°C for at least 2 h to allow re-expression of the vSAg (*see* **Note 6**).

3.3. Flow Cytometric Detection of vSAg7

1. Wash the spleen cells and/or transfectants in HBSS, count, and resuspend cells at final concentration of $0.5–1 \times 10^7$ cell/mL in wash buffer.
2. Add 50 µL of cells to one well of a V-well microtiter plate.
3. Add 10 µL of flow cytometry blocking solution.
4. Add 30 µL of the 3× concentrated primary antibodies. Appropriate controls include the use of secondary reagents alone, splenocytes from strains that do not express the vSAg, and peptides that block the binding of the antibodies, when available (*see* **Note 7**).

5. Incubate the microtiter plates at 4°C for 30–60 min.
6. Centrifuge at 600–1000g for 3–5 min using a swinging bucket centrifuge outfitted with adapters that will accept microtiter plates.
7. Remove the supernatant by "flicking" the plate above the sink. If this is done appropriately, few cells will be lost.
8. Loosen cells remaining in the wells by brief agitation (10–20 s) on a laboratory vortex device equipped with an adapter that will accept microtitre plates. Add 150 µL wash buffer using a multichannel pipettor.
9. Wash the cells by repeating **steps 5–7** two times.
10. After the final wash, add 30 µL of wash bufffer to the wells containing cells and residual buffer, followed by 10 µL secondary detection reagents, or direct fluorochrome coupled antibody conjugates (at 5× concentration). Incubate at 4°C for for 30–60 min.
11. Wash cells once by repeating **steps 5–7**.
12. Resuspend cells in 0.2–0.5 mL wash buffer prior to analysis.
13. Analyze on a flow cytometer. Use forward- and side-scatter parameters to gate on the viable cell population, and adjust gain on the appropriate detectors using the cells incubated with the secondary reagents only to establish baseline fluorescence. Collect a minimum of 10,000 gated events. vSAg expression is generally quite low on normal B cells, although most large B-cell blasts should demonstrate some vSAg fluorescence.

An example of vSAg7 detection on transfectants and on LPS activated B cells is shown in **Fig. 1**. vSAg expression was readily detectable on the transfectant CHIE/S7, but surface expression is typically very low, although detectable, on LPS treated B cells. It is thus essential that appropriate control reagents be used to demonstrate antibody specificity.

Fig. 1. (*see opposite page*) Detection of vSAg7 and class II IE^k on CHO transfectants, and on B-cell blasts. (**A**) Detection of vSAg7 on CHIE/S7. The antibody VS7 (*15*) was biotinylated and used to detect the vSAg. Baseline fluorescence is shown, as determined using the secondary reagent streptavidin phycoerythrin alone (2° only), or VS7 that had been pre-incubated with the cognate synthetic peptide (Ab + peptide). Mean fluorescence values of the cells, indicated by the horizontal marker, were 13.3 for secondary only control, 34.8 for VS7 antibody, and 14.2 for antibody plus peptide. (**B**) Forward-scatter profile of unactivated (– LPS) or activated splenocytes (+ LPS) obtained from a DBA/2J mouse. This

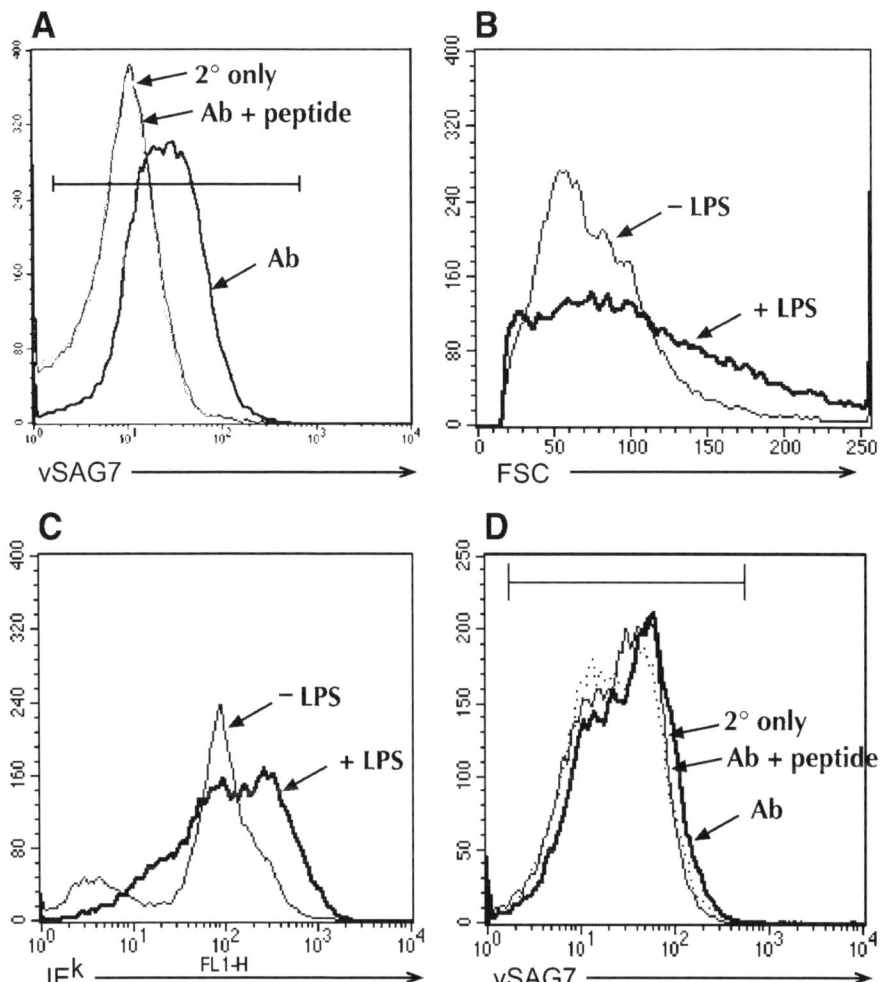

Fig. 1. (*continued*) analysis demonstrates that LPS treatment effectively induced B-cell blasts. Most of the cells that exhibited increased forward scatter were shown to be B cells using a B cell-specific marker (not shown). (**C**) Surface expression of class IE^k on LPS-treated, and untreated, DBA/2J splenocytes. Note that class II MHC expression is elevated on LPS treated cells. (**D**) Expression of vSAg7 on DBA/2J B-cell blasts. Gating was performed on the B cell blasts using forward- and side-scatter gates and vSAg7 was detected as described in (A) Mean fluorescence values of the cells indicated by the horizontal marker were 33.9 and 35.2 for secondary only and antibody plus peptide controls, respectively, and 44.0 for antibody-stained cells.

4. Notes

1. The choice of strain used to detect a particular vSAg is dependent on the proviruses that are carried by inbred mouse strains. For example, the MMTV7 provirus is carried by DBA/2 and other strains (e.g., CBA/J, BALB/D2), but not BALB/c. Alternatively, vSAG6, encoded by MMTV6, is carried by BALB/c, C3H/HeJ, and others (*see* **ref. 10** for a detailed study of the strain distribution of MMT proviruses). Moreover, the level of functional expression of different vSAgs of proviral origin may be quite variable *(22)*. It is critical, therefore, that the appropriate mouse strains be chosen for study.

2. Several MHC class II antibodies are available commercially that can be used for flow cytometry, including 14-4-4S (BD Pharmingen). The antibody 14-4-4S recognizes strains that express IEk or IEd. Note that mouse strains that express some class II haplotypes do not express the IE antigen (e.g., H-2^b, H-2^q, H-2^s). The use of the class II antibodies is not necessary, but the antibodies serve as a good controls for staining technique. Class II surface expression levels are typically one to two logs higher than vSAg staining.

3. Fc receptor blocking reagents are required to inhibit binding of antibodies to Fc receptors on target cells.

4. LPS is required to induce expression of vSAgs on B cells. IL-4 has also be shown to increase the levels of functional vSAgs on B cells *(22)*, so it may be possible to enhance vSAg expression by treatment with both LPS and IL-4.

5. CHIE/S7 is a CHO cell transfectant that expresses the MHC class II protein IE^k and vSAg7 *(5)*. Transfection was performed using expression plasmids that encoded resistance to the antibiotics puromycin (for class II IE^k) and G418 sulfate (for vSAg7).

6. Surface expression of vSAg7, and presumably other vSAgs, is highly sensitive to trypsin, but normal levels of vSAg expression can be restored within 2 h by culture in complete media at 37°C in polypropylene test tubes (to prevent re-attachment). The test tubes containing the cells should be agitated periodically to keep the cells in suspension during the incubation.

7. vSAg expression on the surface of B cells is typically quite low relative to other lymphocyte markers, so it is imperative that one or more specificity controls be used. These include competitor peptides (for peptide-specific antibodies), irrelevant isotype-matched antibodies,

secondary reagent-only controls, and mouse strains that lack expression of the particular vSAg under consideration (*see* **Note 1**).

Acknowledgments

This work was supported by US Public Health Service grant CA69710-02. The author also acknowledges the use of the Wadsworth Center Immunology Core Facility.

References

1. Acha-Orbea, H. and MacDonald, H. R. (1995) Superantigens of mouse mammary tumor virus. *Ann. Rev. Immunol.* **13,** 459–486.
2. Acha-Orbea, H., Finke, D., Attinger, A., Schmid, S., Wehrli, N., Vacheron, S., et al. (1999) Interplays between mouse mammary tumor virus and the cellular and humoral immune response. *Immunol. Rev.* **168,** 287–303.
3. Festenstein, H. (1973) Immunogenetic and biological aspects of in vitro lymphocyte allotransformation (MLR) in the mouse. *Transplant. Rev.* **15,** 62–88.
4. Winslow, G. M., Kappler, J., and Marrack, P. (1997) Structural features of MMTV superantigens. In *Superantigens: Structure, Biology, and Relevance to Human Disease.* Leung, D., Huber, B., and Schlieverts, P. (eds.), Marcel Dekker, New York, NY, pp. 37–60.
5. Mix, D. and Winslow, G.M. (1996) Proteolytic processing activates a viral superantigen. *J. Exp. Med.* **184,** 1549–1554.
6. Winslow, G. M., Cronin, T., Mix, D., and Reilly, M. (1998) Redundant proteolytic activation of a viral superantigen. *Mol. Immunol.* **35,** 897–903.
7. Denis, F., Shoukry, N. H., Delcourt, M., Thibodeau, J., Labrecque, N., McGrath, H., et al. (2000) Alternative proteolytic processing of mouse mammary tumor virus superantigens. *J. Virol.* **74,** 3067–3073.
8. Reilly, M., Mix, D., Reilly, A. A., Ye, Y. Y., and Winslow, G. M. (2000) Intercellular transfer of a soluble viral superantigen. *J. Virol.* **74,** 8262–8267.
9. Beutner, U., McLellan, B., Kraus, E., and Huber, B. T. (1996) Lack of MMTV superantigen presentation in MHC class II -deficient mice. *Cell. Immunol.* **168,** 141–147.

10. Scherer, M. T., Ignatowicz, L., Winslow, G., Kappler, J. W., and Marrack, P. (1993) Superantigens: bacterial and viral proteins that manipulate the immune system. *Ann. Rev. Cell Biol.* **9**, 101–128.

11. Acha-Orbea, H., Held, W., Waanders, G. A., Shakhov, A. N., Scarpellino, L., Lees, R. K., and MacDonald, H. R. (1993) Exogenous and endogenous mouse mammary tumor virus superantigens. *Immunol. Rev.* **131**, 5–25.

12. Held, W., Shakhov, A. N., Waanders, G., Scarpellino, L., Luethy, R., Kraehenbuhl, J.-P., et al. (1992) An exogenous mouse mammary tumor virus with properties of Mls-1ᵃ. *J. Exp. Med.* **175**, 1623–1633.

13. Ardavín, C., Waanders, G., Ferrero, I., Anju`ere, F., Acha-Orbea, H., and MacDonald, H.R. (1996) Expression and presentation of endogenous mouse mammary tumor virus superantigens by thymic and splenic dendritic cells and B cells. *J. Immunol.* **157**, 2798–2794.

14. Webb, S. R. and Sprent, J. (1990) Induction of neonatal tolerance to Mlsᵃ antigens by CD8⁺ T cells. *Science* **248**, 1643–1646.

15. Winslow, G. M., Scherer, M. T., Kappler, J. W., and Marrack, P. (1992) Detection and biochemical characterization of the mouse mammary tumor virus 7 superantigen (Mls-1ᵃ). *Cell* **71**, 719–730.

16. Winslow, G. M., Marrack, P., and Kappler, J. W. (1994) Processing and Major Histocompatibility Complex binding of the MTV7 superantigen. *Immunity* **1**, 23–34.

17. Krummenacher, C. and Diggelmann, H. (1993) The mouse mammary tumor virus long terminal repeat encodes a 47 kDa glycoprotein with a short half-life in mammalian cells. *Mol. Immunol.* **30**, 1151–1157.

18. McMahon, C. W., Bogatzki, L. Y., and Pullen, A. M. (1997) Mouse mammary tumor virus superantigens require N-linked glycosylation for effective presentation to T cells. *Virology* **228**, 161–170.

19. Subramanyam, M., McLellan, B., Labrecque, N., Sekaly, R., and Huber, B. T. (1993) Presentation of the Mls-1 superantigen by human HLA class II molecules to murine T cells. *J. Immunol.* **151**, 2538–2545.

20. Mishell, R. I. and Dutton, R. W. (1967) Immunization of dissociated spleen cell cultures from normal mice. *J. Exp. Med.* **126**, 423–442.

21. Mohan, N., Mottershead, D., Subramanyam, M., Beutner, U. and Huber, B. T. (1993) Production and characterization of an Mls-1-specific monoclonal antibody. *J. Exp. Med.* **177**, 351–358.

22. Gollub, K. J. and Palmer, E. (1991) The physiologic expression of two superantigens in the BDF₁ mouse. *J. Immunol.* **147**, 2447–2454.

4

Spectrophotometric Methods for the Determination of Superantigen Structure and Stability

Anders Cavallin, Karin Petersson, and Göran Forsberg

1. Introduction

An important characteristic of superantigens (SAgs) is their high structural stability. For instance, it is well known that staphylococcal enterotoxins are stable enough to traverse the stomach while retaining their biological activity. Despite this high stability, structural flexibility may be a very important parameter to control their functions such as recognition of certain T-cell receptor (TCR) V_β-chains. The biological properties of SAgs are well-characterized and most residues involved in their functional interactions such as binding to major histocompatibility complex (MHC) class II or TCR have been identified *(1)*. However, those residues often also have important roles for their stability *(2)*.

Here we describe methods to study stability properties of staphylococcal superantigens. The examples given were performed using recombinant SEA, SEB, and SEH. The three-dimensional structures of these proteins have been solved *(3–5)*, facilitating the interpretation of these results.

Thermal and chemical denaturation methods have been used to study the impact of some functionally important residues or regions

From: *Methods in Molecular Biology, vol. 214: Superantigen Protocols*
Edited by: T. Krakauer © Humana Press Inc., Totowa, NJ

on SAg stability. In these studies staphylococcal enterotoxin A and E (SEA and SEE) were most extensively studied *(2)*. These superantigens are sequentially homologous, with more than 80% sequence identity, but they differ substantially in stability as well as in biological properties *(6)*. The stability of these two SAgs as well as SEA/E chimeras were investigated. One major finding was that the MHC class II binding regions, and the Zn^{2+} binding site in particular, are very important for the high structural stability of these SAgs. Modifications in the TCR-binding region substantially affect the molecular conformation indicating more flexibility in this region. In addition to SEA and SEE, the recently discovered SEH is thermally stabilized by Zn^{2+} *(see* **Fig. 1**). In analogy with SEA, SEH has been shown to bind a zinc ion and to be dependent on the zinc ion when interacting with MHC class II *(7,8)*. The thermodynamic impact of Zn^{2+} binding to SEA has been more detailly studied by microcalorimetry *(9)*. In the case of SEB, no stabilizing effect was detected *(see* **Fig. 1**), which was expected since SEB has not been shown to bind zinc ions *(10)*.

The methods described here are thermal denaturation monitored using UV spectrophotometry and guanidine-HCl induced denaturation monitored using circular dichroism (CD). The first is a fast and easy way to determine the melting point(s) of proteins in different buffers measuring the absorbance of the aromatic amino acids phenylalanine, tyrosine, and tryptophan. At denaturation the protein conformation is changed, exposing or hiding these residues, yielding a measurable shift in the protein spectra.

Near UV CD also measures changes in the environment of the aromatic amino acid residues, whereas far UV CD yields information regarding the secondary structure. This means that using CD the conformational changes in tertiary and secondary structure during unfolding can be studied separately. For a more detailed description *see* **refs.** *(11,12)*.

A method often used to study folding or unfolding of proteins is based on tryptophan fluorescence. However, unlike many other proteins SEA and SEE are less suitable for this method. The reason is that during denaturation their fluorescence properties are not significantly altered (data not shown).

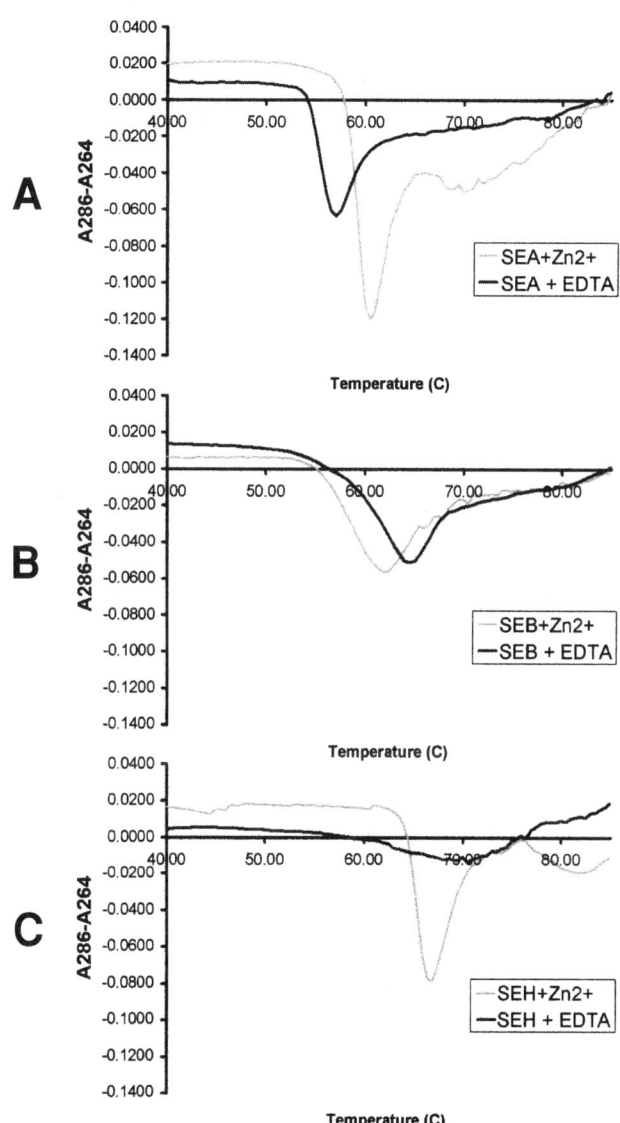

Fig. 1. Thermal denaturations of SEA (**A**), SEB (**B**), and SEH (**C**) monitored using UV spectrophotometry, by measuring the absorbance difference $A_{286}–A_{264}$. The melting point is here defined as the minima of the first derivative of the UV-trace. Both SEA and SEH are stabilized by addition of Zn^{2+}, but this effect is not seen for SEB. The melting points were 55.4°C and 59.2°C for SEA, 62.2°C and 59.0°C for SEB, 62.6°C and 65.4°C for SEH, with EDTA and Zn^{2+}, respectively.

2. Materials

All superantigens used were expressed as secreted products in *Escherichia coli* and purified using ion exchange chromatography at Active Biotech Research AB (Lund, Sweden). The final purity of the products was more than 90% as determined using sodium dodecyl sulfate polyacrylamide gel electrophoresis (SDS-PAGE) *(2,13)* (*see* **Notes 1–3**).

2.1. UV-Monitored Thermal Denaturation

1. A buffer with controlled ionic strength, for example 20 mM phosphate or Tris-buffered saline (TBS) (25 mM Tris, 150 mM NaCl) adjusted to the desired pH. At neutral pH, bound metal ions stabilize the structure, while at pH below 6.0, this effect is less pronounced. Use freshly prepared buffers.
2. Dialysis membranes or PD-10 columns (Amersham Pharmacia Biotech, Uppsala, Sweden) are used for buffer exchanges.
3. A quartz cuvet with 1.0-cm pathlength, preferably with a width of 1 cm as well to provide space for the stirring magnet.
4. A UV diode array spectrophotometer with a heating cell and a magnetic stirrer, for example, the HP8453 (Hewlett-Packard, Waldbronn, Germany).

2.2. CD-Monitored Guanidine-Induced Denaturation

1. A buffer with low absorbance at 220 nm; for example, 20 mM phosphate buffer.
2. 6 M Guanidine-HCl of more than 99% purity (Sigma, Sigma-Aldrich Chemie Gmbh, Germany).
3. Dialysis membranes or PD-10 columns (Amersham Pharmacia Biotech) are used for buffer exchanges.
4. Two quartz cuvet with pathlengths of 1.0 cm, and 0.1 cm, respectively, designed for CD measurements.
5. An instrument capable of measuring far (220 nm) and near (280 nm) CD signals, for example the Jasco J720 (Japan Spectroscopic Co. Ltd., Hachioji City, Japan).
6. A UV spectrophotometer capable of measuring A_{280} and A_{220}, for example the HP8453 (Hewlett-Packard).

3. Methods

3.1. Thermal Denaturation Monitored Using UV Spectrophotometry

The main advantage with thermal denaturations is that only one sample is needed for the whole procedure, and the protein can be kept in an environment that is constant throughout the denaturation procedure, which is not the case with chemical denaturation. The information obtained regarding changes in structural conformation at denaturation is, however, limited when monitored using UV spectrophotometry compared to CD (*see* **Note 4**).

The procedure described utilizes a HP 8453 UV diode-array spectrophotometer with a heating cell, magnetic stirrer (Hewlett-Packard) and associated software (UV-visible Chemstation revision A.02.04a). The method can be extended to any instrument with similar properties.

1. Transfer the superantigen to a TBS or phosphate buffer using dialysis or a PD-10 column. Then dilute the protein to a concentration of 0.1 mg/mL using the same buffer (*see* **Note 5**).
2. Wash the cuvet with 6 *M* Guanidine-HCl and rinse thoroughly with Millipore water (*see* **Note 2**).
3. Carry out baseline correction with the buffer used in **step 1**.
4. Add the sample to the washed and dried cuvet and insert the stirring magnet.
5. For the thermal denaturation monitor the absorbance difference A_{286}-A_{264} between the start and end temperature in steps of 0.5°C with at least 30 s incubation at each temperature. Suitable start and end temperatures are 40°C and 80°C, respectively (*see* **Note 6**).
6. Discard the sample in a bottle containing 1 *M* NaOH to destroy any remaining superantigen and wash the cuvet with 6 *M* Guanidine-HCl followed by a thorough water rinse.

3.2. Guanidine-HCl-Induced Denaturation Monitored Using CD

Chemical denaturations require more material than thermal denaturations, especially when monitored using CD, which require high protein concentrations because usually one sample has to be prepared for each measurement. However, the advantage of using this method is that changes in structural conformation during denaturation can be more detailly studied with the possibility to monitor secondary and tertiary structure unfolding separately (*see* **Note 7**).

The procedure described utilizes a Jasco J720 (Japan Spectroscopic Co. Ltd.). The method can be extended to any instrument with similar properties. The optimal protein concentration yields an absorbance at the measured wavelength of approx 1. For far UV CD this means an A_{220} of approx 1 and for near UV CD an A_{280} of similar magnitude. This corresponds to approx 0.2 mg/mL and 0.8 mg/mL superantigen for far and near UV CD, respectively.

1. Transfer the superantigen to 20 m*M* phosphate buffer, pH 6.0 using dialysis or a PD-10 column (Pharmacia Biotech). Then concentrate the protein to at least 5 mg/mL using ultrafiltration, for example Centriprep10 (Amicon).
2. Make a protein sample series with an increasing amount of guanidine-HCl by using two stock solutions, the first containing 20 m*M* phosphate buffer, pH 6.0, and the second 8 *M* guanidine-HCl in 20 m*M* phosphate, pH 6.0. Use the protein concentrations recommended above (*see* **Note 8**).
3. Incubate each sample for at least 1 h before measuring the CD signal.
4. Discard each sample in a bottle containing 1 *M* NaOH to destroy any remaining superantigen and wash the cuvet with water between each measurement. After measuring all the samples also wash the cuvet with 6 *M* guanidine-HCl followed by a thorough water rinse.
5. For each guanidine concentration used also measure the background signal using a sample not containing superantigen. This signal should then be withdrawn from the raw CD signal.

When analyzing the CD signals, corrections should be made for concentration differences between samples. For proteins with a high sequence identity as well as similar size and composition of aromatic residues, an approximation is to divide the sample CD signal, after subtraction of the blank CD signal, with the protein concentration. Thereby, samples with different protein concentrations can be compared. In **Fig. 2**, the denaturation curves for SEA

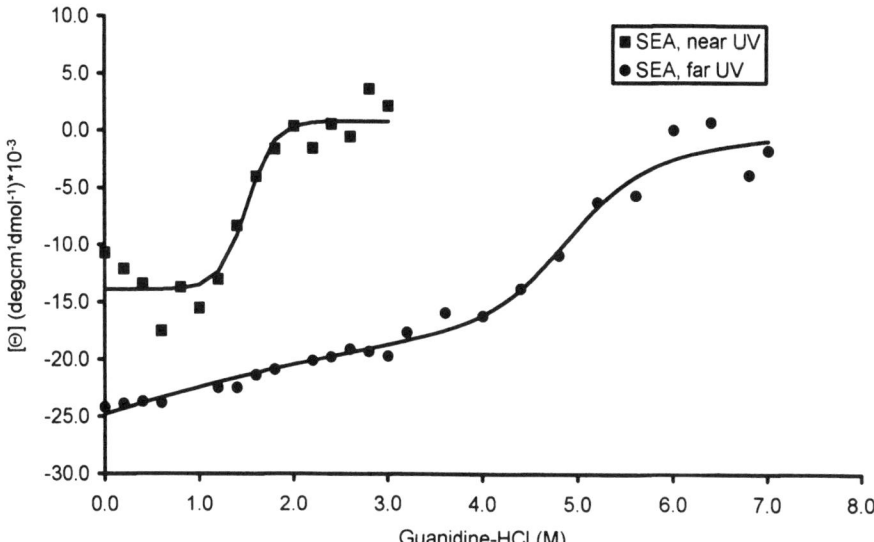

Fig. 2. Far (●) and near (■) UV CD signal, resulting from the secondary and tertiary structure respectively, for SEA in different concentrations of Guanidine-HCl. As the tertiary and secondary structure of the protein unfold, the respective CD signal approach zero.

measured using far (secondary structure) and near (tertiary structure) UV CD is shown. The tertiary structure is lost much earlier than the secondary structure.

4. Notes

1. SAgs are very stable proteins and can therefore be stored for long periods of time. It is preferable to store them in low salt buffer, such as 150 mM sodium acetate at pH 4.5–6.0 and –80°C, but they can be stored at 4°C for 2 d.
2. Most importantly, when working with the very toxic SAgs use protective gloves at all times. Also, all superantigen-containing samples should be disposed of in 1 M NaOH. Cuvets, being sensitive to NaOH, should be washed with 6 M Guanidine-HCl, which also removes any remaining precipitate.
3. For accurate results the purity of the protein analyzed should be at

least 90% determined using SDS-PAGE and/or isoelectric focusing (IEF).

4. During thermal unfolding of SAgs the protein usually precipitates, i.e., the unfolding is not reversible. Because of this, thermodynamic data for the unfolding cannot be obtained. However, adding for example subdenaturing concentrations of guanidine-HCl, less than 1 *M* (*see* **Fig. 2**) can prevent the precipitation. Alternatively, the unfolded SAg is soluble below pH 4.0.

5. Because the SAgs easily aggregate during thermal unfolding the protein concentration should not be too high (≈ 5 μM) as the protein may precipitate before it is fully unfolded, yielding a lowered melting point.

6. When selecting the wavelengths to use when monitoring denaturations, the spectra for native, denatured, and any existing transition states should be studied. Wavelengths should be chosen to obtain the highest possible signal change during transitions. For the SAgs examined here, A_{286}-A_{264} was optimal.

7. Guanidine-induced denaturations demand substantially more work as well as more material due to the large amount of samples needed. However, the additional information obtained when studying tertiary and secondary structure unfolding separately using near and far UV CD often makes it worth the effort.

8. CD-monitored thermal denaturations of SAgs are not recommended because of the aforementioned precipitation and the high concentrations necessary for CD. The consequence is a very noisy signal at denaturation. Also, UV-monitored, guanidine-induced denaturations are not recommended *(11)*.

References

1. Papegeorgiou, A. C. and Acharya, K. R. (2000) Microbial superantigens: from structure to function. *Trends Microbiol.* **8,** 369–375.
2. Cavallin, A., Arozenius, H., Kristensson, K., Antonsson, P., Otzen, D. E., Björk, P., and Forsberg, G. (2000) The spectral and thermodynamical Properties of Staphylococcal enterotoxin A, E and variants suggest that structural modifications are important to control function. *J. Biol. Chem.* **275,** 1665–1672.
3. Schad, E. M., Zaitseva, I., Zaitsev, V. N., Dohlsten, M., Kalland, T.,

Schlievert, P. M., et al. (1995) Crystal structure of the superantigen staphylococcal enterotoxin type A. *EMBO J.* **14**, 3292–3301.

4. Papageorgiou, A. C, Tranter, H. S, and Achraya, K. R (1998) Crystal structure of microbial superantigen staphylococcal enetrotoxin B at 1.5 Å resolutiom: implications for superantigan recognition by MHC class II molecules and T cells receptors. *J. Mol. Biol.* **277**, 61–79.

5. Håkansson, M., Petersson, K., Nilsson, H., Forsberg, G., Björk, P., Antonsson, P., and Svensson, L. A. (2000) The crystal structure of staphylococcal enterotoxin H: implications for binding properties to MHC class II and TCR molecules. *J. Mol. Biol.* **302**, 527–537.

6. Antonsson, P., Wingren, A. G., Hansson, J., Kalland, T., Varga, M., and Dohlsten, M. (1997) Functional characterisation of the interaction between the superantigen staphylococcal enterotoxin A and the TCR. *J. Immunol.* **158**, 4245–4251.

7. Petersson, K., Håkansson, M., Nilsson, H., Forsberg, G., Svensson, A. L., Liljas, A., and Walse, B. (2001) Crystal structure of a superantigen in complex with MHC class II shows zinc and peptide dependence. *EMBO J.* **20**, 3306–3312.

8. Abrahmsén, L., Dohlsten, M., Segrén, S., Björk, P., Jonsson, E., and Kalland, T. (1995) Characterization of two distinct MHC class II binding sites in the superantigen staphylococcal enterotoxin A. *EMBO J.* **14**, 2978–2986.

9. Sundström, M., Hallén, D., Svensson, A., Schad, E., Dohlsten, M., and Abrahmsén, L. (1996) The co-crystal structure of staphylococcal enterotoxin type A with Zn^{2+} at 2.7 Å resolution. *J. Biol. Chem.* **271**, 32,212–32,216.

10. Jardetzky, T. S., Brown, J. H., Gorga, J. C., Stern, L. J., Urban, R. G., Chi, Y., et al. (1994) Three-dimensional structure of a human class II histocompatibility molecule complexed with a superantigen. *Nature* **368**, 711–718.

11. Pace, C. N., Shirley, B. A., and Thomson, J. A. (1989) In: *Protein Structure: A Practical Approach* (Creighton, T. E., ed.), IRL Press, Oxford, UK, pp. 311–313.

12. Schmid, F. X. (1989) In: *Protein Structure: A Practical Approach* (Creighton, T. E., ed.), IRL Press, Oxford, UK, pp. 251–285.

13. Nilsson, H., Björk, P., Dohlsten, M., and Antonsson, P. (1999) Staphylococcal enterotoxin H displays unique MHC class II-binding properties. *J. Immunol.* **163**, 6686–6693.

5

Binding Kinetics of Superantigen with TCR and MHC Class II

S. Munir Alam and Nicholas R. J. Gascoigne

1. Introduction

There are several key differences between the nature of interactions of a T-cell receptor (TCR) with a conventional MHC-peptide complex and a bacterial superantigen (SAg). Apart from being powerful T-cell mitogens, these SAgs do not require antigen processing, they interact with the V_β region of TCR and their binding sites lie outside the peptide-binding groove of the major histocompatibility complex (MHC) class II molecule *(1–5)*. The plasticity of TCR binding to MHC-peptide complex has been appreciated only recently from crystal structures of TCR-MHC complex *(6,7)*. However, the breadth of response to different MHC-peptide ligands is limited, whereas bacterial SAgs commonly interact with several V_β elements. This results largely from the fact that much of the contact is with main-chain atoms instead of side-chain residues of TCR V_β *(5,8,9)*. Taking into account these differences and particularly the strength of the SAg effect on T-cell activation, it was reasonable to predict that bacterial SAgs would interact with higher affinity and that they would also show different binding kinetics.

From: *Methods in Molecular Biology, vol. 214: Superantigen Protocols*
Edited by: T. Krakauer © Humana Press Inc., Totowa, NJ

Currently, the preferred instrument for the measurement of receptor-ligand binding affinity and kinetics is the BIAcore™ *(10)*. This real-time biosensor technology developed by BIAcore AB (Uppsala, Sweden), monitors protein-protein interactions using an optical detection principle based on surface plasmon resonance (SPR). The SPR response reflects a change in mass concentration at the detector surface as receptor-ligand complexes form or dissociate. This allows monitoring of all phases in a protein-protein binding sequence, such that binding affinity and kinetics can be readily derived *(11,12)*. The sensor chip, which is a glass slide with a thin layer of gold on one side, is the signal transducer of this continuous flow-detection system. The gold film is covered with a covalently bound dextran matrix on which proteins can be immobilized and binding interactions between immobilized ligand and soluble analyte can be monitored in real time. Advantages of this technology are that it requires relatively small amounts of sample and that no labeling of proteins is necessary. Recent studies have increasingly relied on BIAcore for measuring binding affinity and kinetics of TCR binding to its ligands and have provided very useful information regarding T-cell recognition (reviewed in **refs.** *13,14*). BIAcore binding studies revealed that TCR-MHC binding is relatively weak, with rapid dissociation of the ligand from the TCR ($t_{1/2}$ = 2–25 s). Quite surprisingly, SAgs also bind to TCR with weak affinity *(15–20)* and their binding affinity for class II molecules is at best of moderate strength *(15,17–23)*. In the case of *Staphylococcus aureus* A (SEA), which has higher affinity for class II when compared to *Staphyloccus aureus* B (SEB), the binding is Zn^{2+}-dependent and the affinity is strongly influenced by the peptide bound to class II *(24,25)*. Some of these peptides may even lower the binding affinity *(25)*. These individual weak interactions between each component of the ternary complex, thus fail to account for the strong mitogenic effect of SAgs. It is, however, likely that these individual interactions may be stabilized during the formation of the trimolecular complex between SAgs, TCR, and class II molecules. A synergistic binding effect was observed when SEB premixed with class II was flowed over an immobilized TCR surface *(15)*. In our study using SEA, we were able to quantitatively analyze the kinetics of the binding interactions between SEA, TCR, and class II *(19)*. Mariuzza and colleagues obtained similar results with SEC3 *(20)*. We found that there was a cooperative effect of interactions during the formation of the trimolecular complex and that this effect enhances the stability of the complex. Interestingly, this enhancement brings the strength of the interactions with SAgs close to those measured for TCR binding to conventional MHC-peptide complex *(19,20)*. This is an important finding as it suggests that even the most potent stimulators of T cells interact with an affinity that is optimum for T-cell activation. Here we describe the methodology used in setting up BIAcore binding experiments for quantitatively measuring the affinity and kinetics of the interactions between a bacterial SAg, SEA, a soluble TCR, and mouse class II, I-E^k.

2. Materials

2.1. Soluble TCR and MHC Proteins

In this study, we have used the 2B4 TCR, which recognizes peptide residues 81–104 from pigeon cytochrome c complexed to the murine MHC class II, I-E^k *(26–28)*. Soluble TCR and MHC proteins can be prepared using various expression systems. Several of these expression systems, which include bacterial, yeast (*Pichia pastoris*), and *Drosophila*, have been found to yield appreciable quantities of soluble TCR proteins in our hands *(19,29,30)*, although no technique has worked well for all TCRs. The 2B4 TCR described here was expressed using *Pichia pastoris* expression vectors pPIC9 and pPIC9K (Invitrogen, San Diego, CA) *(19)*.

The methods for the production of active MHC class II proteins in soluble forms are highly reproducible. Currently, the most commonly used methods include insect cell expression of truncated proteins *(31,32)* and *Escherichia coli* expression and refolding from inclusion bodies *(33)*. In the study described here, soluble Class II I-E^k proteins were purified from Triton X-100 lysates of CH1 (H-2^k) B lymphoma cells by affinity chromatography on a 14-4-4S MAb column *(34)*. Purified I-E^k proteins were stored at –20°C at 50–200 μg/mL in 0.25% n-octylglucoside, 10 mM Tris, pH 8.0, and 150 mM NaCl.

2.2. Bacterial superantigens

Staphylococcus aureus enterotoxin A (SEA) was purchased from Toxin Technology (Sarasota, FL) as lyophilized protein from PBS solution. The SEA was dissolved in deionized water at 0.5–1.0 mg/mL.

2.3. Fast Performance Liquid Chromatography (FPLC)

1. Size-exclusion chromatography columns: Superdex HR200; Superdex 75 (Pharmacia, Uppsala, Sweden)
2. Equilibration buffer: PBS, pH 7.4, containing 150 mM NaCl.
3. An FPLC system (Pharmacia, Uppsala, Sweden) or similar.

2.4. BIAcore Reagents

All these are available from BIAcore, Inc. (Piscataway, NJ).

1. Flow buffer: PBS, pH 7.4, containing 150 mM NaCl, 0.005% surfactant P20.
2. Immobilization solution: Immobilization solutions are available from BIAcore, Inc. as a coupling kit. The amine coupling kit contains the following reagents:
   a. NHS (0.1 M N-hydroxysuccinimide);
   b. EDC (0.1 M N-ethyl-N'-[3-diethylaminopropyl] carboidimide); and
   c. A deactivation solution (1 M ethanolamine, pH 8.5).
3. Immobilization buffer: 10 mM Na-Acetate, pH 4.5.
4. Sensor chip: Research grade CM-5 sensor chip.

2.5. Protein Quantification

1. Bio-Rad protein assay dye.
2. BSA (1 mg/mL) in deionized water is used as stock solution for preparation of a protein estimation standard curve.

2.6. Equipment

1. BIAcore instrument: BIAcore™ 2000 or BIAcore™ 3000 (BIAcore AB, Uppsala, Sweden). Both the 2000 and 3000 machines are PC driven and by using reagent delivery robotics allow complete walkaway automation.

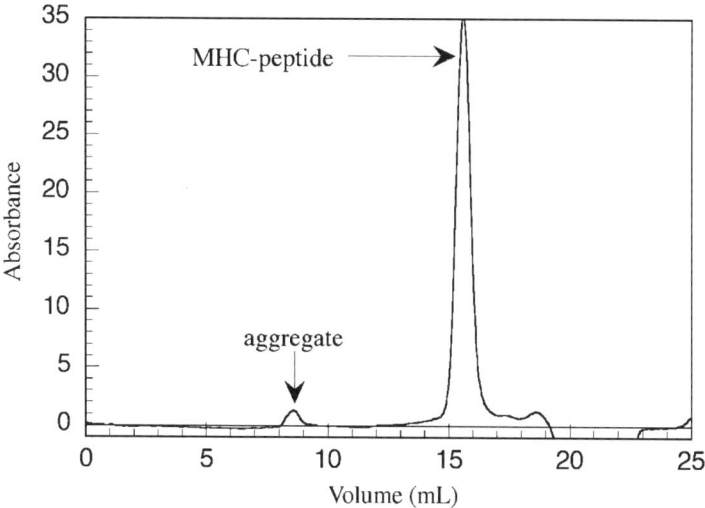

Fig. 1. Removal of protein aggregates by gel-filtration chromatography. Prior to running protein samples on the BIAcore, protein aggregates are removed by gel filtration chromatography. The figure illustrates a typical example of separation of protein aggregates upon FPLC gel-filtration chromatography and using a Superdex HR-200 (Pharmacia) column. A 0.5 mL of soluble MHC-peptide protein sample was injected into the column and the aggregate and the MHC-peptide peaks were eluted at a flow rate of 0.7 mL/min.

2. A Pentium-based desktop computer installed with BIAevaluation 3.0 software (BIAcore AB) for data analysis.

3. Method

3.1. FPLC Purification of Proteins

It is essential that highly purified proteins be used for BIAcore binding kinetics determination. All purified proteins to be used in BIAcore binding assays are first subjected to size-exclusion chromatography. This step is important in removing protein aggregates that might be present and is performed as close to the BIAcore binding assays as possible, preferably the same day or the night before. Although larger aggregates tend not to bind, dimers or trimers can cause potential complexity in the nature of binding. A representative example of separation of aggregates from active MHC proteins over a Superdex HR200 column is shown in **Fig.1**.

3.2. Immobilization of Proteins

In all BIAcore measurements of biomolecular interaction, a protein is selected for coupling to the sensor chip ('the ligand'), while the binding partner ('the analyte') is pumped over the ligand surface. The first step in SPR measurements of protein-protein binding interaction studies is, therefore, the selection of immobilization chemistry. For most protein ligands, the most commonly used coupling chemistry is "amine coupling." However, it is advisable to use other, more favorable chemistry, which may allow a site-directed approach to surface immobilization (*see* **Note 1**). Some of these coupling chemistries (e.g, thiol, aldehyde, biotin-streptavidin) are useful in preparing a more homogenous ligand surface and often help to avoid some of the pitfalls of amine coupling. Other experimental design and analysis considerations, such as mass transport, rebinding, and so on, are highlighted in a recent issue of this series *(35)*.

For studying the trimolecular interactions between TCR, MHC, and SEA, we found that immobilization of MHC proteins gave the best results. Before ligand immobilization using amine coupling, the optimal pH for the coupling buffer must be determined using a "preconcentration step." In most cases, the appropriate pH for the coupling buffer is the highest pH (generally between pH 3.5–6.0) at which there are effective electrostatic interactions between the $-COO^-$ groups on the dextran molecules on the surface of the chip and the $-NH_2^+$ group on the ligand protein. For I-E^k proteins, the best preconcentration effect was achieved at pH 4.5 (*see* **Note 2**) and the immobilization was, therefore, carried out in 10 mM Acetate, pH 4.5.

The following scheme for immobilization may be carried out either on a manual mode or by running a programmed method (*see* **Table 1** and **Note 2**) using the methods automation feature available

Table 1
A Typical BIAcore Method File for Immobilization
of MHC Proteins Using Amine-Coupling Chemistry

DEFINE APROG MHC immob			
FLOW	5		
FLOWPATH	1,2		
TRANSFER	R2A1	R2A3	NHS
TRANSFER	R2A2	R2A3	EDC
MIX	R2A3	110	NHS/EDC
INJECT	R2A3	35	NHS/EDC
-b RPOINT			Baseline
FLOWPATH 2			
INJECT	R2B1	15	Ligand
FLOWPATH 1,2			
RPOINT 1			Immobilized ligand
INJECT R2C1	35		ethanolamine
RPOINT2			Final RU immobilized
END			
MAIN			
FLOWCELL	1,2,3,4		
APROG MHC immob			
Append Standby			
END			

with the BIAcore control software. Details of running sensorgram and method files are available in the BIAcore Applications manual. All of the procedures described here are best performed using a BIAcore 2000 or 3000 instrument. Both of these instruments allow multi-channel flow and detection of binding signals.

3.2.1. Protocol I

1. Dilute stock MHC proteins to 100–300 μg/mL in coupling buffer (10 mM Na-Acetate buffer, pH 4.5).
2. Set flow rate at 5 μL/min.
3. INJECT 35 μL of the NHS/EDC mix (1:1).

4. INJECT 10 µL of MHC proteins in coupling buffer from **step 1** above. Roughly allow coupling of 2000–3000 Response Unit (RU) of MHC proteins (*see* **Note 3**). The amount of proteins to be immobilized can be controlled using the "IF-THEN" command in the method file.
5. INJECT 35 µL of 1 *M* ethanolamine. This will block all the remaining reactive ester groups on the sensor surface.
6. Record amount of immobilized MHC ligand. This is the difference in RU between the final level and the initial baseline RU. There might be some baseline drift during the post immobilization period and it is customary to flow buffer for sometime to allow the baseline to stabilize.

Prepare a blank surface by following **steps 2–5**, and by replacing injection of MHC proteins with flow buffer in **step 4**, **Subheading 3.2.1.** Ideally, the first flow cell (Flow cell 1) is designated the blank surface as it allows in-line reference subtraction of bulk response from an adjacent test surface (Flow cell 2). Alternatively, a method program can be run. It is essentially an automated method program for **steps 1–6** outlined earlier. A typical example of an immobilization method file is given in **Table 1**.

3.3. SPR Binding Analysis

3.3.1. Binding Kinetics of SEA to Immobilized MHC Class II

The formation of a tri-molecular complex between SEA, MHC class II, and TCR, can be followed in a step-wise manner, with the first step being the formation of the SEA-class II complex. SEA binds to class II with a moderate affinity *(24,25)*, and the formation of SEA-class II complexes can be monitored on the BIAcore by injecting SEA over a class II-immobilized sensor surface.

3.3.1.1. PROTOCOL II

1. Run sensorgram on Flow cell 1 (blank) and 2 (MHC) at a flow rate of 10 µL/min.
2. INJECT 15 µL of SEA at 10 µg/mL.
3. Allow sufficient time for buffer flow (usually 300–600 s) in order to get baseline back to the initial baseline level in **step 6**, **Subheading 3.2.1.** *See* **Note 4** on regeneration.

4. Examine binding curve (FC 2-1) for the interactions between SEA and MHC class II. The subtracted curve (FC 2-1) should show specific binding signal.

Having shown that the MHC surface specifically binds to SEA, the next step is to determine the rate constants for the binding of SEA to class II. The following are important considerations for setting up of a kinetics measurement:

a. Dissociation phase. Use of KINJECT command consumes slightly more sample but allows a noise-free dissociation phase, the length of which is pre-determined. This is important for an accurate measurement of off-rate, particularly for interactions that display fast kinetics. In our example of SEA binding to immobilized I-E^k, 300–400 s of dissociation time was selected, during which >90% of the SEA-class II complex had dissociated.

b. Association phase. The length of association should be long enough to allow binding to reach steady-state. This is a reflection of the binding affinity and the amount of ligand immobilized. Generally, a low ligand surface is preferred for kinetics measurement and the exact level of immobilization needs to be experimentally predetermined. Steady-state binding allows determination of equilibrium dissociation constant (K_{eq}) in addition to the apparent K_d that can be calculated from on- and off-rates.

c. Range of analyte protein concentration. A good rule-of-thumb is to use a range from $0.1–10 \times K_d$. Generally 4 or more concentrations of analyte protein are selected that span this range.

d. In-line reference subtraction may be chosen in the method file by using FLOWPATH 2-1 in the method program. Reference surface may be a blank surface that has been activated and then deactivated with the immobilization solutions. Alternatively, an irrelevant protein surface, which shows no binding to the analyte protein, can also serve as a control.

In our example shown in **Fig. 2A** dose-dependent binding curves were generated by injecting SEA over MHC-immobilized surface at concentrations ranging from 0.5–10 μg/mL.

3.3.2. Binding Kinetics of Soluble TCR to Immobilized SEA and MHC Class II

Rate and equilibrium constants for the interactions between TCR, class II, and SEA can be measured by following the steps described

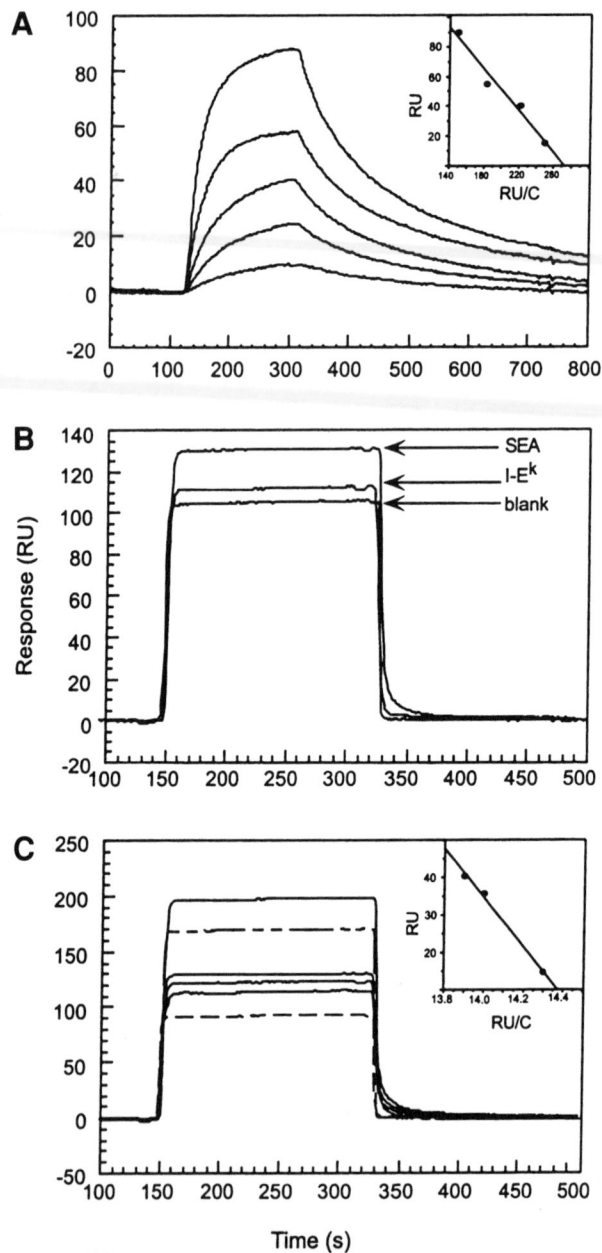

Fig. 2. Binding of a bacterial superantigen, SEA to MHC class II and TCR. In (**A**), by injecting varying concentrations of SEA, a dose-dependent binding of SEA to immobilized MHC class II (I-E^k) was observed. The inset shows a plot of RU vs RU/C, where RU is the binding response

above for SEA-class II binding. The only exception is the nature of the binding kinetics. The 2B4 TCR showed such fast binding kinetics for both SEA and I-E^k that the on-rate could not be reliably measured (*see* **Fig. 2B**) *(19)*. However, for TCR-SEA binding, the off-rate is measurable and the K_{eq} can be measured from steady-state binding data. Assessment of weak binding interactions also require that relatively high concentrations of analyte be injected such that specific binding responses can be calculated after subtraction of bulk or nonspecific binding signal from the control surface (*see* **Note 5**).

3.3.2.1. Protocol III

1. About 500–1000 RU of bacterial toxin (SEA), 2000 RU of class II proteins are immobilized using amine-coupling chemistry and as outlined in **Subheading 3.2.** Include a third adjacent flow cell as a control blank surface (activated and deactivated with immobilization solutions).
2. Inject varying concentrations of TCR proteins (0.4–2.0 μ*M* were used in **Fig. 3**, *see* **Note 5**) over the blank surface and those immobilized with SEA and class II. Owing to fast binding kinetics, there is no requirement for regeneration of the surfaces between each cycle.
3. Analyze binding data for TCR-SEA interactions for K_{eq} measurements.

Fig. 2. (*continued*) at equilibrium and C is the concentration of the injected analyte (SEA). The equilibrium dissociation constant of the binding is calculated from the slope (K_{eq} = -slope) of the scatchard plot. The low-affinity binding of TCR (2B4) to immobilized SEA, I-E^k and a blank surface is demonstrated in the composite curve in (**B**). An injection of 2B4 TCR (1.2 μ*M*) was simultaneously passed over the above surfaces. Binding of SEA to TCR is barely detectable above the bulk response, whereas a higher steady-state binding is observed between SEA and class II. The K_{eq} of the binding of TCR to SEA was calculated by injecting varying concentrations of TCR over the SEA immobilized surface (**C**). Dotted lines show the nonspecific bulk responses generated by flowing TCR over a blank surface. The inset shows the scatchard plot, from which the K_{eq} of TCR-SEA binding was determined. Reproduced with permission from **ref.** *(19)*, copyright 1999, *The American Association of Immunologists*.

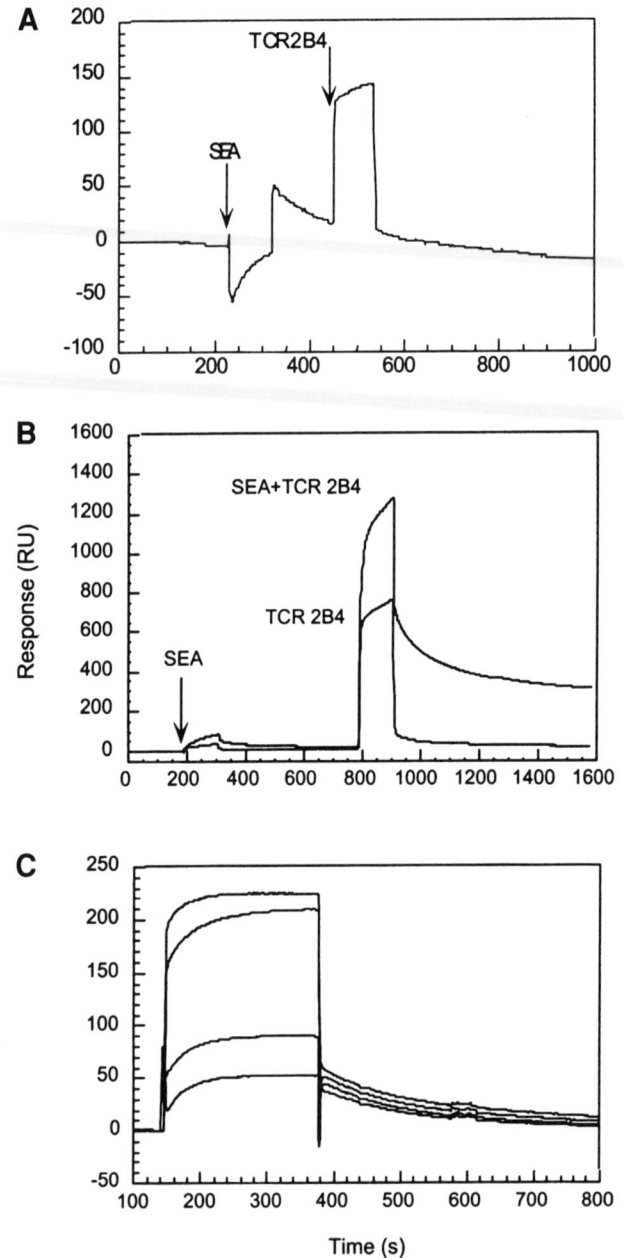

Fig. 3. Formation of the tri-molecular complex between SEA, TCR, and MHC class II. In (**A**), sequential injections of SEA and TCR over immobilized I-E^k fail to create a stable SEA-TCR-class II complex (*see* **Fig. 1**).

3.3.3. SEA-Class II-TCR Trimolecular Complex Formation

Binding of a SAg premixed with soluble class II to immobilized TCR shows a synergistic increase in binding signal *(15,19)*. We also found this to be the best approach in generating a SAg-class II-TCR trimolecular complex *(19)*. In our study with SEA binding to immobilized class II, the SEA-class II complex was relatively short-lived ($t_{1/2}$ = 3 min). Thus, sequential injections of SEA and TCR over a class II surface did not result in the formation of a stable complex and as such no kinetic data could be generated from it (*see* **Fig. 3A**). In contrast, co-injecting TCR and SEA over the class II surface showed higher binding responses and the formation of a much more stable ternary complex (*see* **Fig. 3B**).

3.3.3.1. PROTOCOL IV

1. Inject varying concentrations of TCR (we used 0.4–2.4 μM in **Fig. 3C**) premixed with a constant concentration of SEA (1–5 µg/mL) at 10 µL/min.
2. The length of the injection needs to be optimized for steady-state binding. In our example, a 3-min injection at 10 µL/min was adequate for the binding to reach steady-state (*see* **Fig. 3C**).
3. Analyze data for kinetic and equilibrium constant measurements.

3.4. Analysis of Binding Kinetics

The binding rate and equilibrium constants are generally determined using the BIAevaluation analysis program 3.0 (BIAcore

---

Fig. 3. (*continued*) However in (**B**), mixed injections of SEA (1 µg/mL) and TCR(0.8 μM) over I-E^k surface show higher binding responses and complex binding kinetics when compared to individual binding of SEA and TCR. The binding of SEA to class II is overlayed with its binding to TCR and the binding of TCR to class II is overlayed with those of TCR+SEA. Varying concentrations of TCR (2.4, 2.0, 0.8, and 0.4 μM), mixed with a constant concentration of SEA (1 µg/mL) were injected over a class II immobilized surface (**C**). Reproduced with permission from **ref.** *(19)*, copyright 1999, *The American Association of Immunologists.*

Inc.). The program utilizes a nonlinear curve fitting of the experimental curve to a selected model and the analysis includes an algorithm in which goodness of fit is assessed *(36)*. The program allows the user to select an interaction model based on the known mechanism of interactions between receptor and ligand, if such exists. Model editing is an option and more complex models can also be imported into the program. The reliability of the selected model and the calculated rate constants is based on an assessment of goodness of fit (χ^2 values, residual plots) of the experimental curve to the fitted curve.

3.4.1. SEA-Class II Interactions

Binding of SEA to I-E^k follows the Langmuir model for bimolecular interaction (A + B = AB) and using this model in the nonlinear curve fitting process we found the interaction to be of moderate affinity ($K_d = 0.13$ μM). The apparent K_d is calculated as K_d = off rate/on rate, where the rate constants are derived from the curve fitting process. The binding interactions of SEA to I-E^k show relatively fast on-rate ($k_a = 3.2 \times 10^{-4}$ $M^{-1}s^{-1}$) and a moderately slow off-rate ($k_d = 3.5 \times 10^{-3}$ s^{-1}) *(19)*. The equilibrium constant (K_{eq}) can be measured from a Scatchard plot of RU vs RU/C (-slope = K_{eq}), where RU is the specific response unit at steady state (*see* **Fig. 2A**). The calculated K_{eq} value of 0.32 μM is similar to the dissociation constant measured from rate constants.

3.4.2. SEA-TCR Interactions

The binding of 2B4 TCR to I-E^k, in the absence of the specific cytochrome c peptide, was of extremely low affinity. The fast association could not be reliably measured and the estimation of the dissociation rate indicates that the K_d is likely to be >2 $\times$ 10^{-4} M. This TCR, however, binds to immobilized SEA with a measurable affinity. The binding kinetics was still relatively fast and, as with most weak interactions, we calculated the K_{eq} of 6.9 $\times$ 10^{-5} M for this binding from a Scatchard plot analysis. The TCR, therefore, binds to the bacterial SAg, SEA with a higher affinity than the virtually negligible binding to class II.

3.4.3. SEA-Class II-TCR Ternary Complex

Formation of a ternary complex is a biphasic process and is likely to involve more complex binding interactions. For instance, the first complex may act to initiate and stabilize the formation of the ternary complex. In a two-step process, the formation of the ternary complex may, therefore, be dependent on the stability of the complex formed in the first step. Our initial approach of sequential injection of SEA and TCR produced only transient interactions of the TCR with its ligand (*see* **Fig. 3A**). This binding curve failed to provide any quantitative data for the binding of TCR to SEA-class II complex. When TCR was premixed with SEA, we observed a substantial increase in binding response, indicating the formation of a more stable ternary complex (*see* **Fig. 3B**). As expected, these bi-phasic binding curves failed to provide an acceptable fit to the simple, Langmuir model. Based on the theoretically perceived binding interactions, we, therefore, used a "noncompetitive analyte" binding model to describe the formation of the ternary complex (*see* **Note 6**). This is a two-step model, in which two noncompeting analytes bind to independent sites on the same ligand according to the following scheme:

$$A_1 + B = A_1B; A_2 + A_1B = A_1A_2B$$

The first component (A_1) binds to the immobilized ligand to form a complex A_1B, which is followed by a second step in which another analyte molecule (A_2) binds to form a ternary complex (A_1A_2B) with the existing binary complex. In other words, the first step of this model apparently describes the binding of SEA (A_1) to class II (B) and the second step accounts for the interaction between TCR (A_2) and SEA-class II complex (A_1B), resulting in the formation of the trimolecular complex (A_1A_2B). The curves shown in **Fig. 3C** gave a better fit to this model, showing an acceptable goodness of

Table 2
Kinetic Rate Constants for the Trimolecular Interactions
Among SEA, TCR, and Class II Molecules

Analyte	Ligand	k_{on} $(M^{-1}s^{-1})$	k_{off} (s^{-1})	K_d μM
TCR + SEA	I-E^k	step 1 3.6×10^4	3.5×10^{-3}	0.097
		step 2 4.8×10^3	1.1×10^{-2}	2.27

Adapted with permission from **ref.** *(19)*, copyright 1999, *The American Associaton of Immunologists.*

fit ($\chi^2 = 0.037$). The rate constants derived for the first and faster binding interactions were similar to those calculated for SEA-class II interactions (*see* **Table 2**). This was expected as SEA-class II interactions are of higher affinity. The second step, which apparently describes formation of the ternary complex, gave slower on and off rates (*see* **Table 2**). However, there was an increase in the $t_{1/2}$ of the ternary complex (36.5 s) when compared to TCR-SEA interactions (10.7 s). The binding affinity of the SEA-TCR-class II was calculated to be 2.3×10^{-6} *M*. This affinity is comparable to those measured for TCR-MHC-peptide interactions *(13,14,29,30)*. Thus, like activation of T cells by MHC-peptide ligands, the bacterial SAg SEA interacts with TCR with relatively low affinity, which is stabilized during the formation of the trimolecular complex with class II molecules.

BIAcore analysis has proven very useful for the investigation of interactions between pairs of TCR, MHC class II, and SAgs, and for measurement of the synergistic ternary complex between these three components. Such studies, coupled with X-ray crystallographic structural information has led to a very clear understanding of how binding to the TCR V$_\beta$-region leads T-cell activation by SAgs.

4. Notes

1. Although amine-coupling of proteins is the simplest and most commonly used technique, it may be preferable to use a site-directed coupling chemistry. Amine coupling can give rise to surface het-

erogeneity owing to immobilization of proteins at random sites and this in turn, can give rise to complexity in the binding interactions. The immobilized surface is also much less than active and as such the immobilized level is to be corrected for any loss in activity due to heterogeneous orientation of the ligand. The activity of the ligand surface can be determined by flowing anti-MHC antibodies over it. In comparison to amine-coupling, we have observed at least a twofold increase in activity of immobilized MHC proteins when they were coupled using a site-directed approach like thiol coupling *(27)*. Several specialized sensor chips (NTA for capturing his-tagged proteins, SA for biotinylated proteins) are now available from BIAcore that allow users more choice in their immobilization chemistry.

2. The Wizard program included with the BIAcontrol software 3.0 allows user- friendly set up of method files for immobilization and kinetics experiment.

3. The level of immobilization of a ligand is dependent on the nature of experiment and the binding kinetics. In designing a kinetics experiment, the recommendations are to use a lower level of ligand, generally enough to give about 100–200 RU of binding. In case of low mw ligands, kinetics data can be reliably measured from even lower binding responses. However, higher immobilized level can be used when creating a ligand-capture surface or during determination of sample concentration.

4. Regeneration of surface after each cycle of binding is an important step in a BIAcore experimental design. However, ideal regeneration conditions need to be determined experimentally such that these allow effective disruption of ligand-receptor interactions but at the same time it should not compromise the activity of the ligand surface. Often for weak binding interactions (SEA-TCR, TCR-MHC-peptide) or binding displaying moderately fast kinetics (SEA-class II), regeneration of a ligand surface can be achieved by simply washing the surface with flow buffer *(18,26)*.

5. The kinetics of weak binding interactions requires several considerations. In some cases, the binding kinetics may be too fast to measure on or off rates. In such cases only K_{eq} values can be measured from steady-state binding data. It is important to include a reliable control surface for subtraction of nonspecific signal. In some cases, the specific-to-nonspecific signal may be small (as in TCR-class II binding), and therefore, higher analyte concentrations may be required. Although in our example here, we have used a blank sur-

face for bulk signal subtraction, a more ideal control surface may include an irrelevant protein of similar size and immobilized to the same RU level. A higher flow rate (20 μL/min or higher) is also recommended for resolving specific signal from bulk effect.

6. In general, a complex model is selected only after the simple model fails to provide a good fit or if the proposed mechanism of binding describes a complex mode of interaction. However, it is also important to rule out surface heterogeneity, rebinding, and mass-transport effects as the cause of binding complexity. As pointed out earlier, surface heterogeneity can be resolved by using a different coupling chemistry, while rebinding and mass transport effects can be avoided by using lower immobilization levels and higher flow rates respectively. In our assessment of the formation of a ternary complex, we have used a two-step complex model to describe the interactions between SEA, TCR, and class II. A useful test of such a linked-reaction is to vary the contact time of analyte injections. Shorter injection time will allow only the first step to go to completion and therefore the binding interactions will more closely follow the simple model *(30)*.

Acknowledgments

This work was supported by NIH R01 GM46134 and 39476 to Nicholas R. J. Gascoigne. S. Munir Alam is a recipient of a Special Fellow Award by the Leukemia and Lymphoma Society and a Scientist Development Grant from American Heart Association. This is publication 14152-IMM from The Scripps Research Institute.

References

1. Scherer, M. T., Ignatowicz, L., Winslow, G. M., Kappler, J. W., and Marrack, P. (1993) Superantigens: bacterial and viral proteins that manipulate the immune system *Annu. Rev. Cell Biol.* **9,** 101–128.
2. Gascoigne, N. R. J. (1993) Interaction of the T cell receptor with bacterial superantigens. *Semin. Immunol.* **5,** 13–21.
3. Gascoigne, N. R. J., Alam, S. M., Haarstad, C. A., and Sim, B.-C. (1995) Structural features of T cell receptor recognition of superantigens, in *Bacterial Superantigens: Structure, Function and*

Therapeutic Potential (Thibodeau, J. and Sekaly, R.-P., eds.) R. G. Landes, Austin, TX, pp. 97–112.

4. Lavoie, P. M., Thibodeau, J. Erard, F., and Sekaly, R.-P. (1999) Understanding the mechanism of action of bacterial superantigens from a decade of research. *Immunol. Rev.* **168**, 257–269.

5. Li, H., Llera, A., Malchiodi, E. L., and Mariuzza, R. A. (1999) The structural basis of T cell activation by superantigens. *Annu. Rev. Immunol.* **17**, 435–466.

6. Garcia, K. C., Teyton, L., and Wilson, I. A. (1999) Structural basis of T cell recognition. *Annu. Rev. Immunol.* **17**, 369–397.

7. Reinherz, E. L., Tan, K., Tang, L., Kern, P., Liu, J., Xiong, Y., et al. (1999) The crystal structure of a T cell receptor in complex with peptide and MHC class II. *Science* **286**, 1913–1921.

8. Fields, B. A., Malchiodi, E. L., Li, H., Ysern, X., Stauffcher, C. V., Schlievert, P.M., et al. (1996) Crystal structure of a TCR β chain complexed with a superantigen. *Nature* **384**, 188–192.

9. Li, H., Llera, A., Tsuchiya, D., Leder, L., Ysern, X., Shlievert, P. M., et al. (1998) Three-dimensional structure of the complex between a T cell receptor β chain and the superantigen staphylococcal enterotoxin B. *Immunity* **9**, 807–816.

10. Fivash, M., Towler, E. M., and Fisher, R. J. (1998) BIAcore for macromolecular interactions. *Curr. Opin. Biotechol.* **9**, 97–101.

11. Myszka, D. G. (1997) Kinetic analysis of macromolecular interactions using surface plasmon resonance biosensor. *Curr. Opin. Biotechnol.* **8**, 50–57.

12. Boniface, J. J. and Davis, M. M. (1994) The kinetics of binding of peptide/MHC complexes to T-cell receptors: application of surface plasmon resonance to a low-affinity measurement. *Methods Enzymol.* **6**, 168–176.

13. Davis, M. M., Boniface, J. J., Reich, Z., Lyons, D., Hampl, J., and Arden, B. (1998) Ligand recognition by αβ T cell receptors. *Annu. Rev. Immunol.* **16**, 523–534.

14. Gascoigne, N. R. J., Zal, T., and Alam, S. M. (2001) T-cell receptor binding kinetics in T-cell development and activation. *Exp. Rev. Mol. Med.* 12 February, http://www-ermm.cbcu.cam.ac.uk/01002502h.htm

15. Seth, A., Stern, L. J., Ottenhoff, T. H., Engel, I., Owen, M. J., Lamb, J. R., et al. (1994) Binary and ternary complexes between T-cell receptor, class II MHC and superantigen in vitro. *Nature* **369**, 324–327.

16. Malchiodi, E. L., Eisenstein, E., Fields, B. A., Ohlendorf, D. H., Schlievert, P. M., Karjalainen, K., and Mariuzza, R. A. (1995) Superantigen binding to a T cell receptor β chain of known structure. *J. Exp. Med.* **187,** 823–833.

17. Khandekar, S. S., Brauer, J., Naylor, J. W., Chang, H.-C., Kern, P., Newomb, J. R., et al. (1997) Affinity and kinetics of the interactions between an αβ T cell receptor and its superantigen and class II-MHC/ peptide ligands. *Mol. Immunol.* **6,** 493–503.

18. Leder, L., Llera, A., Lavoie, P. M., Lebedeva, M. I., Li, H., Sekaly, R.-P., et al. (1998) A mutational analysis of the binding of Staphylo-coccal enterotoxins B and C3 to the T cell receptor β chain and major histocompatibility complex class II. *J. Exp. Med.* **187,** 823–833.

19. Redpath, S., Alam, S. M., Lin, C., O'Rourke, A. M., and Gascoigne, N. R. J. (1999) Cutting Edge: Trimolecular interaction of TCR with MHC class II and bacterial superantigen shows a similar affinity to MHC:peptide ligands. *J. Immunol.* **163,** 6–10.

20. Andersen, P. S., Lavoie, P. M., Sekaly, R.-P., Churchill, H., Kranz, D. M., Schlievert, P. M., et al. (1999) Role of the T cell receptor α chain in stabilizing TCR-superantigen-MHC class II complexes. *Immunity* **10,** 473–483.

21. Fraser, J. D. (1989) High affinity binding of staphylococcal entero-toxins A and B to HLA-DR. *Nature* **339,** 221–223.

22. Mollick, J. A., Cook, R. G., and Rich, R. R. (1989) Class II MHC molecules are specific receptors for Staphylococcus enterotoxin A. *Science* **244,** 817–820.

23. Fisher, H., Dohlstein, M., Lindvall, M., Sjogren, H.-O., and Carlsson, R. (1989) Binding of Staphylococcal enterotoxin A to HLA-DR on B cell lines. *J. Immunol.* **142,** 3151–3157.

24. Hudson, K. R., Tiedemann, R. E., Urban, R. G., Lowe, S. C., Strominger, J. L., Fraser, J. D. (1995) Staphylococcal enterotoxin A has two cooperative binding sites on major histocompatibility complex class II. *J. Exp. Med.* **182,** 711–720.

25. Kozono, H., Parker, D., White, J., Marrack, P., and Kappler, J. (1995) Multiple binding sites for bacterial superantigens on soluble class II MHC molecules. *Immunity* **3,** 187–196.

26. Hedrick, S. M., Matis, L. A., Hecht, T. T., Samelson, L. E., Longo, D. L., Heber-Katz, E., and Schwartz, R. H. (1982) The fine specificity of antigen and Ia determinant recognition by T cell hybridoma clones specific for pigeon cytochrome c. *Cell* **30,** 141–152.

27. Chien, Y., Gascoigne, N. R. J., Kavaler, J., Lee, N. E., and Davis, M. M. (1984) Somatic recombination in a murine T-cell receptor gene. *Nature* **309,** 322–326.
28. Becker, D. M., Patten, P., Chien, Y., Yokota, T., Eshhar, Z., Giedlin, M., et al. (1985) Variability and repertoire size of T-cell receptor Vα gene segments. *Nature* **317,** 430–434.
29. Alam, S. M., Travers, P. J., Wung, J., Nasholds, W., Redpath, S., Jameson, S. C., and Gascoigne, N. R. J. (1996) T cell receptor affinity and thymocyte positive selection. *Nature* **381,** 616–620.
30. Alam, S. M., Davies, M., Nasholds, W., Jameson, S. C., Hogquist, K., Gascoigne, N. R. J., and Travers, P. J. (1999) Qualitative and quantitative differences in T-cell receptor binding kinetics for agonist and antagonist ligands. *Immunity* **10,** 227–237.
31. Stern, L. J. and Wiley, D. C. (1992) The human class II MHC protein HLA-DR1 assembles as empty alpha beta heterodimers in the absence of antigenic peptide. *Cell* **68,** 465–477.
32. Scott, C. A., Garcia, K. C., Carbone, F. R., Wilson, I. A., and Teyton, L. (1996) Role of chain pairing for the production of functional soluble IA major histocompatibility complex class II molecules. *J. Exp. Med.* **183,** 2087–2095.
33. Altman, J. D., Reay, P. A., and Davis, M. M. (1993). Formation of functional class II MHC/peptide complexes from subunits produced in *E. coli. Proc. Natl. Acad. Sci. USA* **89,** 12, 117–121.
34. O'Rourke, A. M. and Lasam, M. C. (1995) Murine CD4⁺ T cells undergo TCR-activated adhesion to extracellular matrix proteins but not to non-antigenic MHC class II proteins. *J. Immunol.* **155,** 3839–3846.
35. Masson, L., Mazza, A., and De Crescenzo, G. (2000) Determination of affinity and kinetic rate constants using surface plasmon resonance, in *Methods in Molecular Biology, vol.145: Bacterial Toxins: Methods and Protocols.* (Holst, O., ed.) Humana Press, Totowa, NJ, pp. 189–201.
36. O'Shannessy, D. J. (1994) Determination of kinetic rate and equilibrium binding constants for macromolecular interactions: a critique of the surface plasmon resonance literature. *Curr. Opin. Biotechnol.* **5,** 65–71.

6

Directed Evolution of T-Cell Receptors for Binding Superantigens

Hywyn R. O. Churchill and David M. Kranz

1. Introduction

A T-cell recognizes two major classes of antigens. Binding of the $\alpha\beta$ T-cell receptor (TCR) to an intracellularly-processed peptide antigen in the context of a major histocompatibility complex (pMHC) provides for the specificity of a cell-mediated immune response. However, this normal antigen recognition event can be circumvented by bacterial and viral proteins called superantigens (SAgs) *(1)*. These unprocessed antigens bind to and thereby cross-link the variable region of the TCR β chain (V_β) with a class II pMHC product, resulting in stimulation of a large subset of T cells. This nonspecific immune response results in detrimental inflammatory reactions, T-cell deletion, and/or T-cell anergy *(2,3)*.

Many structural and biological studies have focused on the SAgs of the *Staphylococcus aureus* bacterium, which have been associated with food poisoning and toxic shock syndrome *(2,4)*. *S. aureus* enterotoxins B and C3 (SEB and SEC3) activate T cells through binding to the V_β TCR with low affinity (140 and 3 μM, respectively) *(4,5)*. However, stabilization of the TCR:SE:pMHC ternary complex through the association of the V_α TCR chain and pMHC

From: *Methods in Molecular Biology, vol. 214: Superantigen Protocols*
Edited by: T. Krakauer © Humana Press Inc., Totowa, NJ

may compensate for this low-affinity interaction *(6)*. The interactions among the entire ternary complex approximate affinities of standard TCR:pMHC interactions *(7,8)*. Recently, we performed alanine scanning mutagenesis to define the functional contribution of V_β TCR residues to SEC3 recognition *(9)*. Based on the finding that selected combinations of alanine substitutions could increase SEC3 binding up to fivefold, we proposed that engineering yet higher-affinity forms of a soluble V_β TCR may serve to block the T cell:SE interaction. To this end, a suitable method of performing directed evolution would be valuable in the identification of mutant V_β TCRs that act as antagonists of SE-mediated T-cell activation.

Phage display has frequently been employed as a technique for affinity maturation of antibodies *(10)*. However, with one exception *(11)*, phage display of TCRs has been problematic. Recently, an alternative system termed yeast surface display has been developed *(12)*. Yeast exhibit protein-folding and post-translational modification mechanisms that are similar to higher organisms (namely mice and humans) and hence yeast display could provide a system for engineering the TCR. In this regard, yeast surface display has recently been used in conjunction with fluorescence-activated cell sorting (FACS) to isolate stabilized and affinity-matured TCRs *(13–17)*. A previous review has described the method of yeast display for protein engineering *(18)*. In this chapter, we describe the use of yeast surface display to screen TCR V_β libraries mutated in contact regions of the V_β TCR:SE complex *(19,20)*. Yeast-cell populations showing increased binding to SEB and SEC3 were selected by flow cytometric sorting and individual yeast clones expressing high-affinity TCR were evaluated for binding SEB and SEC3. The approach provides a high throughput system for the discovery of high-affinity antagonists of superantigen-mediated diseases.

2. Materials

1. Yeast surface display plasmid pCT202. The yeast surface display is based on the **a**-agglutinin cell-cell adhesion system as previously described *(12)*. Features of the expression plasmid include a nine-

residue hemagglutinin (HA) epitope tag and the AGA2 open reading frame downstream of the galactose-inducible promoter *GAL1-10*. The ampicillin resistance gene encoded in the pCR-Script vector (Stratagene) backbone provides for selection in *E. coli*, and the *TRP1* gene serves as the yeast selection marker in the absence of tryptophan. A modified yeast display vector (pYD1) is now available from Invitrogen.

2. *Pwo* DNA polymerase : 5 U/µL, supplied with 10X reaction buffer (Boehringer-Mannheim).

3. dNTPs : 100 mM (Novagen).

4. Restriction endonucleases *Bgl*II, *Bsa*I, and *Nhe*I (New England Biolabs).

5. T4 DNA ligase (New England Biolabs).

6. Electromax DH10B (Gibco-BRL). Electrocompetent *E. coli* strain with the genotype F⁻ *mcr*A Δ(*mrr-hsd*RMS-*mcr*BC) φ80d*lac*Z ΔM15 Δ*lac*X74 *deo*R *rec*A1 *end*A1 *ara*Δ139D(*ara,leu*)7697 *gal*U *gal*K 1⁻ *rps*L *nup*G.

7. Luria Broth containing 100 µg/mL ampicillin (LB-amp).

8. Miniprep DNA Kit (Qiagen).

9. SD-CAA growth medium for yeast: 2% (v/v) glucose, 5% (v/v) casamino acids (trp⁻), 6.7% (v/v) yeast nitrogen base, 100 mM sodium phosphate, pH 6.0.

10. SG-CAA expression medium for yeast: 2% (v/v) galactose replaces glucose in SD-CAA medium. 50 µg/mL kanamycin (Sigma) is added as an antibiotic.

11. *Saccharomyces cerevisiae* strain BJ5465 (MAT **a** *ura3-52 trp1 leu2Δ1 his3Δ200 pep4::HIS2 prb1Δ1.6R can1 GAL (pIU211:URA3)* containing a chromosomally integrated Aga1 open reading frame controlled by the *GAL1-10* promoter (EBY100).

12. Flow Buffer (PBS/BSA): PBS, 0.5% bovine serum albumin (BSA).

13. KJ16 monoclonal antibody (MAb) (rat anti-mouse V$_β$8.2 TCR) *(21)* conjugated to fluorescein (FITC) (1 µg/mL).

14. 9E10 MAb (anti-*c-myc*) raw-ascites fluid (Berkeley Antibody Company).

15. Goat anti-mouse F(ab')$_2$ IgG conjugated to FITC: 1 mg/mL in PBS/BSA (Kirkegaard and PerryLabs).

16. Biotinylated SEB and SEC3: 1 mg/mL in PBS (Toxin Technologies, Inc).

17. Streptavidin-R-phycoerthrin (SAv-PE): 0.5 mg/mL (PharMingen).

3. Methods

3.1. Subcloning and Expression of TCR on the Surface of Yeast

1. The V_β chain of the murine cytotoxic T lymphocyte clone 2C TCR *(22,23)* is amplified by polymerase chain reaction (PCR). A 5' primer complementary to the coding strand is synthesized with a unique *Nhe*I restriction site, and 25 bases that match the 5' end of the gene. A 3' primer complementary to the noncoding strand is synthesized with a unique *Bgl*II restriction site, two stop codons, a 30 base *c-myc* tag sequence, and 25 bases that match the 3' end of the gene. A PCR reaction contains 100 pmol of each primer, 10 ng template DNA (*2C TCR* gene in pUC19 plasmid), 1 μL of *Pwo* DNA polymerase, 10 μL of 10X reaction buffer, 10 μL of 2 m*M* dNTPs, and H_2O to a final volume of 100 μL. The gene is amplified by 25 cycles of melting (94°C, 1 min), annealing (55°C, 1 min), and extension (69°C, 1 min), followed by a finishing cycle (69°C, 10 min) *(24)*. The PCR product is isolated by phenol/chloroform/isoamyl alcohol (PCI) purification *(25)*.

2. PCR product (1 μg) is digested using restriction endonucleases *Nhe*I and *Bgl*II (5 U each) in 100 μL for 1 h at 37°C, and PCI purified.

3. Digested PCR product (10 ng) is inserted into the corresponding restriction sites of the digested plasmid pCT202 (0.1 μg) using T4 DNA ligase (1 μL) in 100 μL for 16 h at 14°C, and PCI purified.

4. The DNA is transformed by electroporation into Electromax DH10B.

5. Plasmids are purified from *E. coli* strain DH10B by DNA miniprep and then transformed by electroporation into the *S. cerevisiae* expression strain EBY100 *(26)*.

6. Electroporated cells are spread onto SD-CAA agar plates that lack tryptophan. A colony of the yeast cells is grown in SD-CAA overnight.

7. At an OD_{600} of 1.0 (approx 1×10^7 cells), the yeast cells are centrifuged at 1000 rpm, and the cells are suspended in 2 mL SG-CAA. Cells are incubated with shaking at 20°C for 24 h to induce surface expression.

8. Surface expression of the stable, properly-folded V_β TCR protein and *c-myc* tag is confirmed by evaluating the binding of KJ16-FITC (1 μg/mL in PBS/BSA) and 9E10-FITC (1:50 dilution in PBS/BSA), respectively, by flow cytometry (*see* **Fig. 1**).

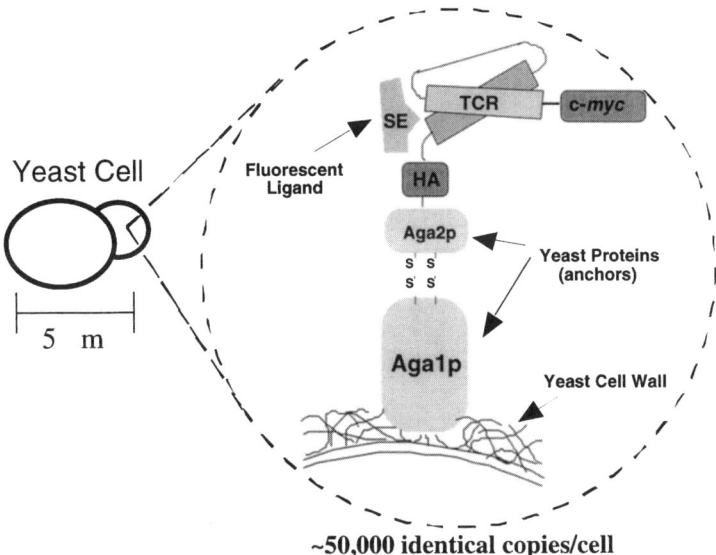

~50,000 identical copies/cell

Fig. 1. Representation of yeast surface display of V_β TCR. The V_β TCR is expressed on the surface of the yeast cell on the C-terminus of the yeast-mating factor AGA-2 and HA epitope tag. Binding of biotinylated SAgs to the surface-displayed V_β TCR followed by SAv:PE as the fluorescent label can be detected by flow cytometry.

3.2. Construction of Mutated TCR Libraries

1. A PCR method is used to mutate codons for three to four amino acids in the V_β TCR/pCT202. A mutagenic primer with degenerate bases (NNS; where N = G, C, A, or T, and S = G or C) at the desired mutation region overlaps with a complementary strand primer to yield exponential PCR (*see* **Note 1**). Each primer encodes a unique *Bsa*I restriction site. The plasmid is amplified by 16 cycles of melting (94°C, 30 s), annealing (55°C, 1 min) and extension (69°C, 14 min), and PCI purified.
2. PCR product (2 µg) is digested at both ends using *Bsa*I restriction endonuclease (10 U) in 100 µL for 1 h at 50°C, and PCI purified.
3. Digested PCR product is ligated using T4 DNA ligase in 100 µL for 16 h at 14°C, and PCI purified.
4. The DNA is transformed by electroporation into Electromax DH10B (5–10 independent transformations yielding a library size of ~10^7).

5. The transformed *E. coli* cells are grown overnight in LB-amp and the plasmid libraries are isolated by DNA miniprep.

6. Yeast cells are transformed with the plasmid preparation containing the mutated V_β TCR DNA libraries by electroporation of pCT202.

7. A 50 µL aliquot of the pooled transformations is plated to determine total number of transformants (10–20 independent transformations of 100 ng each yield library sizes of approx 2×10^6).

8. The remaining electroporated pool is grown in SD-CAA for approx 36 h, to an OD_{600} of 5. The yeast cells are centrifuged at 1000 rpm, and suspended in 20 mL SG-CAA at 20°C for 24 h to induce surface expression.

3.3. Screening and Selection of TCR Libraries Displayed on the Yeast Surface

1. Yeast cells (5×10^7) are suspended in 1 mL PBS/BSA and incubated with various concentrations of biotinylated SEB or SEC3 at 4°C for 1 h.

2. The cells are washed twice with 1 mL PBS/BSA.

3. The cells are incubated with SAv-PE (2.5 µg/mL in PBS/BSA) at 4°C for 1 h.

4. The cells are washed twice with 1 mL PBS/BSA and suspended in 1.0 mL PBS/BSA.

5. Yeast cells were analyzed by flow cytometry and the top 0.5% exhibiting the highest degree of PE fluorescence are collected by flow cytometric sorting.

6. Selected cells (10^4–10^5) are grown in 2 mL SD-CAA.

7. Four successive rounds of sorting and re-growth of selected cells are used to produce distinct populations of positively stained cells (*see* **Fig. 2**) (*see* **Note 2**).

8. The collected cells are grown on SD-CAA agar plates, and individual colonies are evaluated for binding SEB and SEC3 after growth and induction with galactose, as previously described (*see* **Fig. 3**) (*see* **Note 3**).

3.4. Analysis of SAg Binding to Yeast Displayed V_βTCR Mutants

1. Yeast cells (1×10^6) are incubated with 50 µL of biotinylated SEB or SEC3 at various concentrations at 4°C for 1 h.

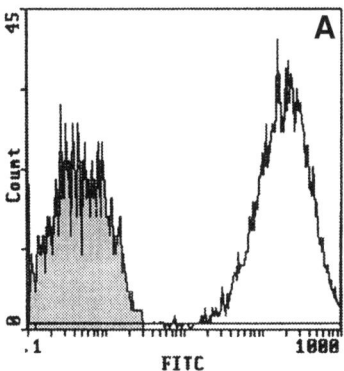 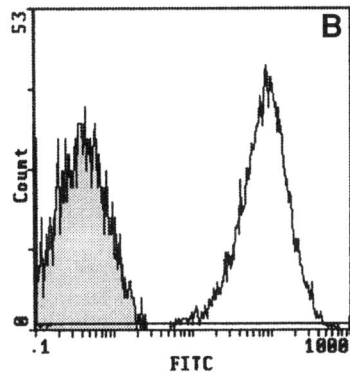

Fig. 2. Flow cytometric analysis of V_β TCR expressed on the surface of yeast. Yeast displaying wild-type V_β TCR were stained with **(A)** KJ16-FITC, and **(B)** 9E10 followed by goat anti-mouse F(ab')$_2$ IgG-FITC. The shaded peak represents the negative (unstained) yeast population, while the unshaded peak represents the population for positive FITC staining. Labeled yeast cells were analyzed on a Coulter Epics XL flow cytometer (Flow Cytometry Facility of the UIUC Biotechnology Center).

2. The cells are washed twice with 250 μL PBS/BSA.
3. The cells are incubated with 50 μL SAv-PE (2.5 μg/mL in PBS/BSA) at 4°C for 1 h.
4. The cells are washed twice with 0.5 mL PBS/BSA and suspended in 1.0 mL PBS/BSA.
5. Yeast cells were analyzed by flow cytometry (*see* **Fig. 4**) (*see* **Note 4**).

4. Notes

1. Introducing variability at additional codons in a gene increases the number of possible independent DNA combinations exponentially. For example, if a single amino acid position of a protein were to include any of the 20 amino acids, the 32 different DNA sequences corresponding to NNS would be required. Because transformation efficiencies readily produce yeast libraries of about 10^7, a maximum of four residues can be changed to cover most permutations ($32^4 \approx 10^6$ different genetic combinations).
2. A method of reiterative selection for mutants, each resulting in an enrichment of those yeast that bear higher-affinity TCRs, is usually

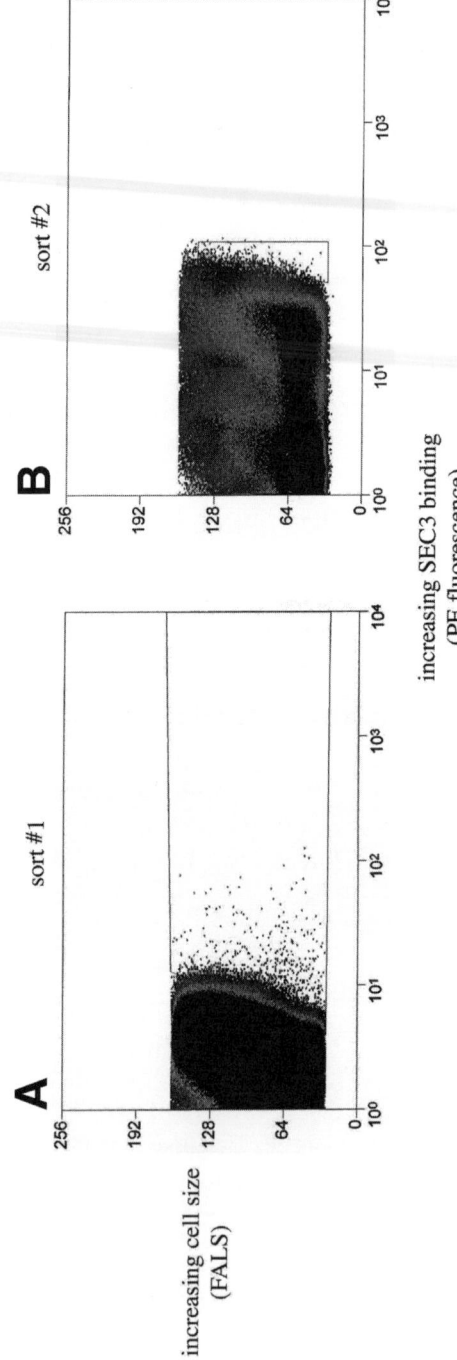

Fig. 3. Cell sorting of a yeast surface displayed mutant V$_\beta$ TCR library. A V$_\beta$ TCR mutant library was labeled with 15 n*M* SEC3-biotin and sorted. The horizontal axis shows the increase in PE fluorescence of the yeast library from the first sort (**A**) to the fourth sort (**B**). Enrichment of positively labeled cells upon iterative sorting results in the formation of a distinct population of cells with the desired binding characteristics. Flow cytometric sorting was performed on a Cytomation MoFlo MLS high speed flow cytometer (Flow Cytometry Facility of the UIUC Biotechnology Center).

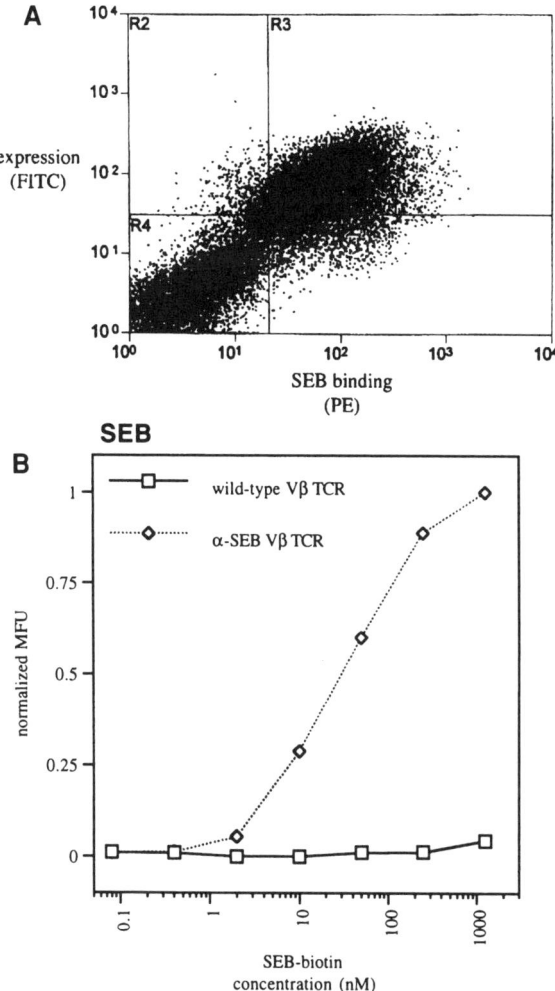

Fig. 4. Flow cytometric analysis of equilibrium SAg binding to V_β TCR mutants displayed on the yeast surface. (**A**) A V_β TCR mutant on the yeast surface was stained with 50 n*M* biotinylated SEB followed by SAv-PE, and 9E10 MAb followed by goat anti-mouse F(ab')$_2$ IgG-FITC. The horizontal axis shows SAg binding to the V_β TCR, and the vertical axis shows expression of the C-terminal *c-myc* epitope tag. (**B**) The same mutant was titrated with varying amounts of biotinylated SEB, followed by SAv-PE. An apparent dissociation constant (K_d) can be determined for the V_β TCR mutant while displayed on the yeast surface, without having to produce soluble protein. The cells were analyzed on a Cytomation MoFlo MLS high speed flow cytometer (Flow Cytometry Facility of the UIUC Biotechnology Center).

necessary. The approach involves several rounds of surface-display induction followed by SEB or SEC3 selection using flow cytometric sorting.

3. As the affinity of the wild-type TCR:SE interactions are micromolar, improvements of over a 1000-fold are necessary to reach nanomolar affinities that might be the target for successful therapeutics. It is possible that a single cycle of mutagenesis will yield only 10- to 100-fold improvements in affinity. Thus it may be desirable to further mutagenize a V_β region(s) selected in the first cycle by targeted mutagenesis of additional residues in the TCR, followed by sorting. Thus, multiple rounds of sorting can be applied to multiple cycles of mutagenesis.

4. One extension of yeast-surface display is the ability to determine the apparent dissociation constant (K_d) of the displayed protein of interest with its ligand by flow cytometry. In the case of V_β TCR:SE interactions, minimal binding of the wild-type V_β TCR can be detected to either SEB or SEC3 *(17)*, consistent with the inherent low binding affinities (140 and 3 μ*M*, respectively) *(5)*. However, after successive rounds of mutagenesis and selection by flow cytometric sorting, the apparent K_d values for the mutant V_β TCR:SE interactions can be determined while the proteins are displayed on the yeast surface, without having to produce soluble protein. This was confirmed by the apparent K_d value of SEC3 binding to a yeast surface-displayed V_β TCR mutant by flow cytometry (6 n*M*), compared to the soluble protein by surface plasmon resonance (7 n*M*) *(17)*.

References

1. Marrack, P. and Kappler, J. (1990) The staphylococcal enterotoxins and their relatives [published erratum appears in Science 1990 Jun 1;248(4959):1066]. *Science* **248,** 705–711.
2. Kotzin, B. L., Leung, D. Y. M., Kappler, J., and Marrack, P. (1993) Superantigens and their potential role in human disease. *Adv. Immunol.* **54,** 99–166.
3. Scherer, M. T., Ignatowicz, L., Winslow, G. M., Kappler, J. W., and Marrack, P. (1993) Superantigens: bacterial and viral proteins that manipulate the immune system. *Annu. Rev. Cell. Biol.* **9,** 101–128.
4. Li, H., Llera, A., Malchiodi, E. L., and Mariuzza, R. A. (1999) The

structural basis of T cell activation by superantigens. *Annu. Rev. Immunol.* **17,** 435–466.

5. Malchiodi, E. L., Eisenstein, E., Fields, B. A., Ohlendorf, D. H., Schlievert, P. M., Karjalainen, K., and Mariuzza, R. A. (1995) Superantigen binding to a T cell receptor b chain of known three-dimensional structure. *J. Exp. Med.* **182,** 1833–1845.

6. Andersen, P. S., Lavoie, P. M., Sekaly, R. P., Churchill, H., Kranz, D. M., Schlievert, P. M., et al. (1999) Role of the T cell receptor alpha chain in stabilizing TCR-superantigen- MHC class II complexes. *Immunity* **10,** 473–483.

7. Eisen, H. N., Sykulev, Y., and Tsomides, T. J. (1996) Antigen-specific T-cell receptors and their reactions with complexes formed by peptides with major histocompatibility complex (MHC) proteins. *Adv. Protein Chem.* **49,** 1–56.

8. Davis, M. M., Boniface, J. J., Reich, Z., Lyons, D., Hampl, J., Arden, B., and Chien, Y. (1998) Ligand recognition by alpha beta T cell receptors. *Annu. Rev. Immunol.* **16,** 523–544.

9. Churchill, H. R., Andersen, P. S., Parke, E. A., Mariuzza, R. A., and Kranz, D. M. (2000) Mapping the energy of superantigen Staphylococcus enterotoxin C3 recognition of an alpha/beta T cell receptor using alanine scanning mutagenesis. *J. Exp. Med.* **191,** 835–846.

10. Winter, G., Griffiths, A. D., Hawkins, R. E., and Hoogenboom, H. R. (1994) Making antibodies by phage display technology. *Annu. Rev. Immunol.* **12,** 433–455.

11. Weidanz, J. A., Card, K. F., Edwards, A., Perlstein, E., and Wong, H. C. (1998) Display of functional αβ single-chain T-cell receptor molecules on the surface of bacteriophage. *J. Immunol. Methods* **221,** 59–76.

12. Boder, E. T. and Wittrup, K. D. (1997) Yeast surface display for screening combinatorial polypeptide libraries. *Nat. Biotechnol.* **15,** 553–557.

13. Kieke, M. C., Shusta, E. V., Boder, E. T., Teyton, L., Wittrup, K. D., and Kranz, D. M. (1999) Selection of functional T cell receptor mutants from a yeast surface-display library. *Proc. Natl. Acad. Sci. USA* **96,** 5651–5656.

14. Shusta, E. V., Kieke, M. C., Parke, E., Kranz, D. M., and Wittrup, K. D. (1999) Yeast polypeptide fusion surface display levels predict thermal stability and soluble secretion efficiency. *J. Mol. Biol.* **292,** 949–956.

15. Holler, P. D., Holman, P. O., Shusta, E. V., O'Herrin, S., Wittrup, K.

D., and Kranz, D. M. (2000) In vitro evolution of a T cell receptor with high affinity for peptide/MHC. *Proc. Natl. Acad. Sci. USA* **97,** 5387–5392.

16. Shusta, E. V., Holler, P. D., Kieke, M. C., Kranz, D. M., and Wittrup, K. D. (2000) Directed evolution of a stable scaffold for T-cell receptor engineering. *Nat. Biotechnol.* **18,** 754–759.

17. Kieke, M. C., Sundberg, E., Shusta, E. V., Mariuzza, R. A., Wittrup, K. D., and Kranz, D. M. (2001) High affinity T cell receptors from yeast display libraries block T cell activation by superantigens. *J. Mol. Biol.* **307,** 1305–1315.

18. Boder, E. T. and Wittrup K. D. (2000) Yeast surface display for directed evolution of protein expression, affinity, and stability. *Methods Enzymol.* **328,** 430–444.

19. Fields, B. A., Malchiodi, E. L., Li, H., Ysern, X., Stauffacher, C. V., Schlievert, P. M., et al. (1996) Crystal structure of a T-cell receptor β-chain complexed with a superantigen. *Nature* **384,** 188–192.

20. Li, H., Llera, A., Tsuchiya, D., Leder, L., Ysern, X., Schlievert, P. M., et al. (1998) Three-dimensional structure of the complex between a T cell receptor beta chain and the superantigen staphylococcal enterotoxin B. *Immunity* **9,** 807–816.

21. Haskins, K., Hannum, C., White, J., Rhoem, N., Kubo, R., Kappler, J., and Marrack, K. (1984) The antigen-specific major histocompatibility complex-restricted receptor on T cells. VI. An antibody to a receptor allotype. *J. Exp. Med.* **160,** 452–471.

22. Kranz, D. M., Sherman, D. H., Sitkovsky, M. V., Pasternack, M. S., and Eisen, H. N. (1984) Immunoprecipitation of cell surface structure of cloned cytotoxic T lymphocytes by clone-specific antisera. *Proc. Natl. Acad. Sci. USA* **81,** 573–577.

23. Soo Hoo, W. F., Lacy, M. J., Denzin, L. K., Voss, E. W. J., Hardman, K. D., and Kranz, D. M. (1992) Characterization of a single-chain T cell receptor expressed in *E. coli. Proc. Natl. Acad. Sci.* **89,** 4759–4763.

24. Coen, D. M. (1994) The polymerase cahin reaction. In: *Current Protocols in Molecular Biology.* (Ausubel, F. M., Brent, R., Kingston, R. E., Moore, D. M., Deisman, J. G., Smith, J. A., and Struhk, K., eds.), J. Wiley and Sons, New York, NY, **Suppl. 16,** pp. 15.1.1–15.1.7.

25. More, D. M. (1994) Preparation of genomic DNA. In: *Current Protocols in Molecular Biology.* (Ausubel, F. M., Brent, R., Kingston, R.

E., Moore, D. M., Deisman, J. G., Smith, J. A., and Struhl, K., eds.), J. Wiley and Sons, New York, NY, **Suppl. 25,** pp. 2.1.1.–2.1.9.

26. Becker, D. M., and Lundbals, V. (1994) Manipulation of yeast genes. In: *Current Protocols in Molecular Biology.* (Ausbel, F. M., Brent, R., Kingston, R. E., Moore, D. M., Deisman, J. G., Smith, J. A., and Struhl, K., eds.), J. Wiley and Sons, New Yrok, NY, **Suppl. 18,** pp. 13.7.1.–13.7.10.

7

Analysis of Superantigen Binding to Soluble T-Cell Receptors

Hywyn R. O. Churchill and David M. Kranz

1. Introduction

The T-cell receptor (TCR) is a membrane-bound, multi-subunit complex that plays a key role in antigen recognition of cell-mediated immunity. The α and β chains of the TCR are extracellular domains that are the primary contact regions for two types of antigens. In conventional T-cell recognition, the $\alpha\beta$ TCR binds to an intracellularly-processed peptide antigen in the context of a major histocompatibility complex (pMHC) on the surface of an antigen-presenting cell (APC), providing for the specificity of an immune response. However, superantigens (SAgs) are unprocessed proteins that circumvent this normal antigen presentation by crosslinking the TCR with a class II pMHC, leading to a nonspecific, polyclonal expansion of T cells *(1)*.

Over the last 10 yrs, many advances in understanding conventional and SAg-mediated immune recognition have been realized through structural studies employing soluble versions of the $\alpha\beta$ TCR. The structures of a β-chain *(2)* and V_α-domain *(3)* confirmed the immunoglobulin-like nature of the TCR. Soon thereafter the structures of two $\alpha\beta$ heterodimers suggested a common diagonal

From: *Methods in Molecular Biology, vol. 214: Superantigen Protocols*
Edited by: T. Krakauer © Humana Press Inc., Totowa, NJ

mode for TCR binding to pMHC *(4,5)*. The first crystal structure of a TCR:SAg complex was solved using a TCR β-chain complexed with *Staphylococcus aureus* enterotoxin C3 (SEC3) *(6)*, and subsequently, the same β-chain complexed with SEB *(7)*. Coupled with biochemical analysis of TCR binding to SE:pMHC complexes, these investigations suggested that SAgs may have evolved to stimulate T cells by mimicing the normal TCR:pMHC interaction *(8–12)*.

Several methods of producing stable, soluble TCRs have been instrumental to the study of TCR:SAg interactions. TCR β-chains employed in the TCR:SAg complexes were expressed in myeloma cells and purified by affinity chromatography *(2)*. These soluble TCR β-chains were also used for biophysical measurements of apparent affinities of the TCR:SAg complexes by sedimentation equlibrium and surface-plasmon resonance *(8)*. Expression of an αβ TCR heterodimer in *Drosophila* cells assisted in defining the role of the TCR α-chain in stabilizing a proposed TCR:SEB:pMHC ternary complex *(10)*. Insect-cell expression was also used to produce the soluble, extracellular domains of αβ TCR DO-11.10 to evaluate its binding to a cell-surface complex of SEB:pMHC *(13)*. The same technology was used to investigate the physical interactions between a class II-restricted TCR D10 and TSST-1, SEB, and SEC2 *(14)*.

There are several drawbacks to the use of mammalian and insect systems for the production of soluble TCRs. The length of time required to obtain stable transfected cell lines that produce functional protein, in addition to more expensive culture reagents, limit the number and quantity of TCRs that can be produced for biochemical and mutagenesis studies. In this chapter, we present methods to produce soluble, SAg-reactive TCRs from *Escherichia coli* rapidly and in large quantities. A $V_\beta V_\alpha$ TCR fused to the *E. coli* protein thioredoxin was constructed *(15)* to facilitate alanine scanning mutagenesis studies of the functional interaction of specific TCR residues for binding SEC3 *(11)*. Also, V_β TCR mutants that bind SEB and SEC3 with high affinity can be produced in yeast or *E. coli* to be evaluated as potential soluble antagonists of

SAg-mediated T-cell activity (*[16]* and unpublished results). As described in Chapter 6, V_β domains can be selected for higher affinity using a yeast display system.

2. Materials

1. ThioFusion expression plasmid pTrxFus (Invitrogen). The plasmid provides for the expression of the V_β-V_α single-chain TCR (scTCR) downstream of the *E. coli* thioredoxin protein (Trx). Protein expression is under the control of the P_L λ phage promoter, which is inhibited by the λ cI repressor. An enterokinase site is encoded between Trx and the TCR for subsequent cleavage, if desired.

2. *Escherichia coli* expression strain GI698. The strain has the genotype F⁻ λ⁻ *lacIq lacPL8 ampC::P_{trp} cI*. The integrated λ cI repressor is under control of the *trp* promoter, allowing for production of the repressor in tryptophan-free medium. The repressor binds the P_L λ phage promoter, thus preventing transcription of the Trx scTCR. Expression is induced by addition of tryptophan (10 mg/mL to a final concentration of 100 µg/mL) to the culture.

3. Growth medium (RM) for *E. coli* GI698. The rich growth medium contains 1X M9 salts (42 m*M* Na$_2$HPO$_4$, 22 m*M* KH$_2$PO$_4$, 8.5 m*M* NaCl, 19 m*M* NH$_4$Cl), 0.2% tryptophan-free casamino acids, 0.5% glucose, 1 m*M* MgCl$_2$, and 50 mg/mL ampicillin.

4. Induction medium (IM) for *E. coli* GI698. The minimal induction medium is similar to RM, except IM contains 0.02% tryptophan-free casamino acids.

5. Prokaryotic expression plasmid pET21b (Novagen). The plasmid provides for the expression of the V_β TCR. Protein expression is under the control of the T7*lac* promoter, which is inhibited by the *lac*I repressor.

6. *Escherichia coli* expression strain BL21 (DE3). The strain has the genotype F⁻ *ompT hsdS_B (r_B⁻m_B⁻) gal dcm* (DE3), and has T7 RNA polymerase integrated into its genome, which is under control of the *lacUV5* promoter. Expression is induced by addition of isopropyl-β-D-thiogalactopyranoside (0.5 *M* IPTG to a final concentration of 1 m*M*, Sigma) to the culture.

7. Growth/expression Luria Broth (LB) for BL21 (DE3). This complete medium contains 1% bacto-peptone, 0.5% yeast extract, 1% NaCl, and 100 µg/mL ampicillin.

8. Osmotic shock buffer : 10 mM Tris-HCl, 2 mM EDTA, pH 8.0.
9. Denaturing buffer: 6 M guanidine-HCl, 20 mM Tris-HCl, at pH 8.0
10. His-Bind (Novagen) and Ni-NTA (Qiagen) affinity gels.
11. TEA refolding buffer: 100 mM Tris-HCl, 2 mM EDTA, 0.4 M arginine (no pH adjustment).
12. Superdex 200 agarose gel (Amersham Pharmacia Biotech).
13. Biotin-labeling buffer : 0.1 M NaCl, 0.1 M NaHCO$_3$ at pH 7.4.
14. Biotin-labeling reagent: biotinamidocaproate N-hydroxysuccinimide ester (Sigma), 10 mg/mL in DMSO.
15. Immulon 2HB 96-Well analytical plates (Dynex Technologies).
16. Blocking/washing solution (PBS/BSA): PBS containing 0.25% bovine serum albumin (BSA) (Sigma) and 0.05% Tween 20 (Sigma).
17. Horseradish peroxidase-streptavidin (HRP-SAv) and tetramethyl-benzidine peroxidase (TMB) substrate (Kirkegaard and Perry).

3. Methods

3.1. Prokaryotic Expression of Single-Chain $\alpha\beta$ T-Cell Receptors

1. The wild-type and alanine-substituted scTCRs of the murine cytotoxic T lymphocyte clone 2C TCR *(17,18)* with a *His$_6$* affinity tag are subcloned by polymerase chain reaction (PCR) into pTrxFus plasmid, as described in Chapter 6, Subheading 3.3.1.
2. The plasmid is transformed by electroporation into *E. coli* GI698, and positive clones are grown in 4 × 2 mL RM at 30°C.
3. The cultures are added to 360 mL RM, and grown at 30°C for 12 h.
4. The culture is subdivided into 6 × 1.5 L IM and grown to an OD$_{600}$ of 0.6 at 30°C (about 3–4 h).
5. Each culture (1.5 L) is induced by adding tryptophan (15 mL, 10 mg/mL), and shaken at 150 rpm at 25°C for 5 h.
6. The bacteria are collected by centrifugation at 5000 rpm.

3.2. Prokaryotic Expression V_β T-Cell Receptors

1. The wild-type and high-affinity mutants of the V_β 2C TCR with a *His6* affinity tag are subcloned by PCR into the pET 21b plasmid, as described in Chapter 6, Subheading 3.3.1.

2. The plasmid is transformed by electroporation into *E. coli* BL21 (DE3), and a positive clone is grown in 4×2 mL LB at 37°C.
3. The cultures are added to 360 mL LB, and grown at 37°C for 12 h.
4. The culture is subdivided into 6×1.5 L LB and grown to an OD_{600} of 0.6–1.0 at 37°C (about 2–3 h).
5. Each culture is induced by adding IPTG (3 mL), and shaken at 200 rpm at 37°C for 3–4 h.
6. The bacteria are collected by centrifugation.

3.3. Isolation and Purification of scTCR and V_β TCR

1. The bacterial pellets are suspended in osmotic shock buffer (180 mL) and passed through a microfluidizer or French press.
2. After washing the inclusion bodies with 0.5% Triton X-100 in osmotic shock buffer (70 mL), the proteins are solubilized in denaturing buffer (70 mL) for 16 h at 4°C.
3. The solubilized proteins are passed over a denaturing nickel affinity column (Novagen, Qiagen), and eluted with 1 M imidazole (20 mL).
4. The proteins are refolded by dialysis in TEA (4×200 mL) at 4°C.
5. The monomeric proteins are purified by size exclusion Superdex 200 gel filtration (*see* **Note 1**).

3.4. Biotinylation of SAgs and TCRs

1. The proteins at approx 100 µg in 100 µL are dialyzed into biotin-labeling buffer at 4°C (*see* **Note 2**).
2. Biotinylation reagent (10 µL per mg of protein) is added.
3. The mixture is incubated for 1 h at 25°C.
4. The mixture is dialyzed into PBS at 4°C (500 mL).

3.5. Binding of Trx-$\alpha\beta$ TCR and V_β TCR to anti-TCR Monoclonal Antibodies

1. Monoclonal anti-V_β antibodies KJ16 *(19)*, F23.1 and F23.2 *(20)* are adsorbed to protein-binding analytical plates by addition of 50 µL of (10 µg/mL in PBS) to each well.
2. The wells are blocked with PBS/BSA (250 µL) for 1 h at room temperature.

3. After washing with PBS/BSA (3 × 250 μL), 100 μL of mutant or wild-type TCR at various concentrations and 50 μL of biotinylated wild-type TCR in PBS/BSA (*see* **Note 3**) are added to the wells and aged for 1 h at room temperature.

4. The wells are washed with PBS/BSA (3 × 250 μL) and binding is detected using HRP-SAv:TMB substrate following the manufacture's protocol. Representative binding curves are shown in **Fig. 1** (*see* **Note 4**).

3.6. Binding of Trx-αβ scTCR and V$_\beta$ TCR to SAgs

1. SAg competition enzyme-linked immunosorbent assays (ELISAs) are performed by adsorption of 50 μL of wild-type scTCR (6 μg/mL in PBS) to each well of an analytical plate.

2. The wells are blocked with PBS/BSA (250 μL) for 1 h at 4°C.

3. After washing with PBS/BSA (3 × 250 μL), 50 μL of mutant or wild-type TCR at various concentrations in PBS/BSA and 50 μL of biotinylated SAgs in PBS/BSA (*see* **Note 5**) are added to the wells and aged for 1 h at 4°C.

4. The wells are washed with PBS/BSA (3 × 250 μL) and binding is detected using HRP-SAv:TMB substrate, following the manufacture's protocol. Representative binding curves of SAg reactivities are shown in **Fig. 2**.

4. Notes

1. Approximately 20% of the Trx-αβ TCR isolated from inclusion bodies is monomeric protein. Size-exclusion gel filtration is necessary to separate the monomer from the protein aggregate. Up to 5 mg of

---

Fig. 1. (*see opposite page*) Reactivity of soluble TCR mutants with anti-V$_\beta$8 antibodies. The relative reactivities of (**A**) Trx-αβ scTCR proteins for V$_\beta$8-specific antibody F23.1 and (**B**) V$_\beta$ TCR proteins for V$_\beta$8-specific antibody KJ16 were evaluated in a competition ELISA format. Various concentrations of wild-type and mutant TCRs were used to inhibit the binding of biotinylated wild-type TCR to each antibody, followed by detection with streptavidin-HRP. The IC$_{50}$ ratios of mutant to wild-type were calculated by linear regression analysis. The average value for each mutant was used as a normalization factor for properly refolded protein.

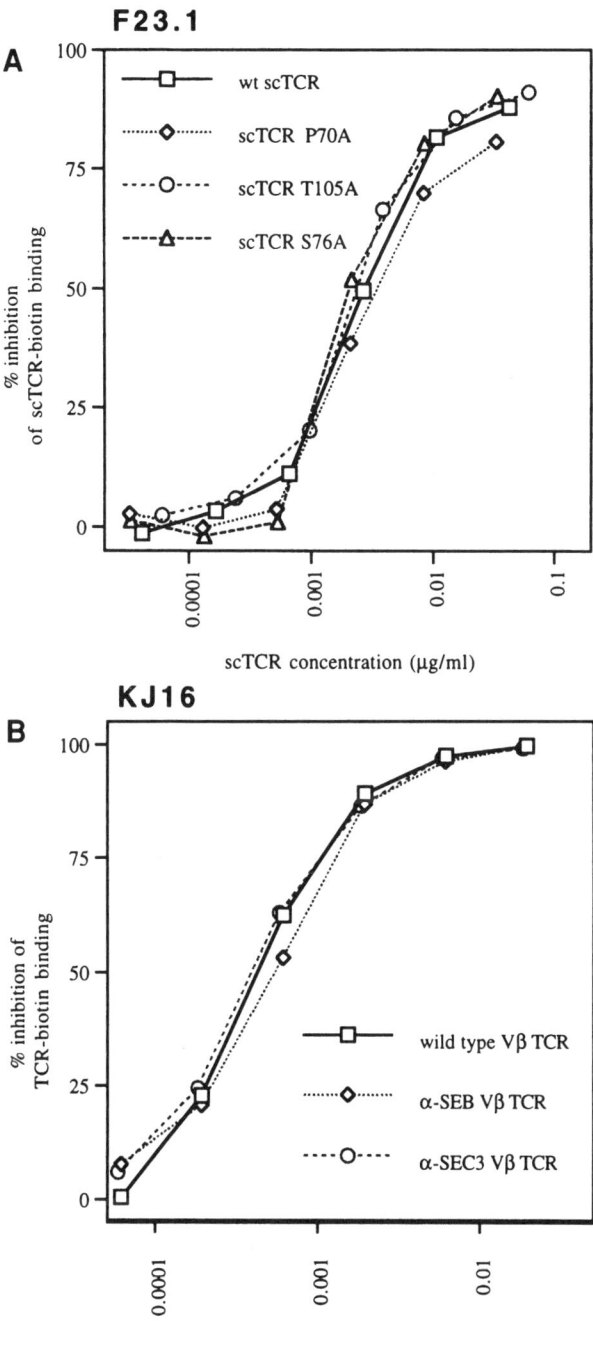

Fig. 1.

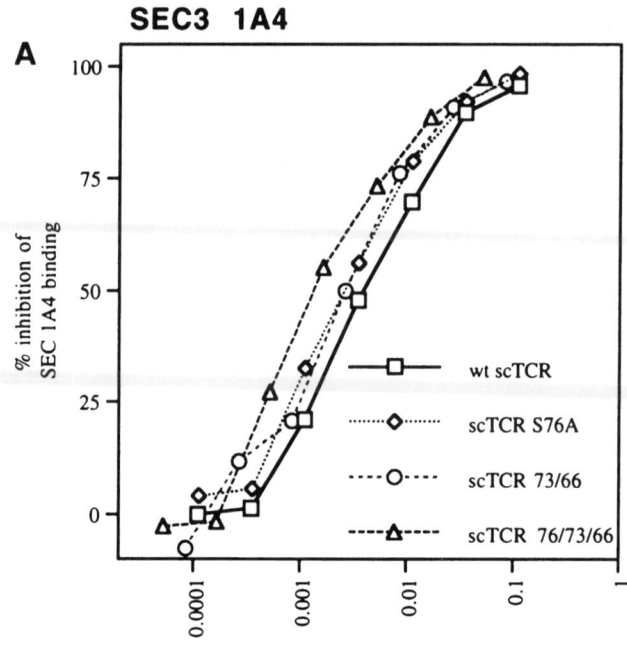

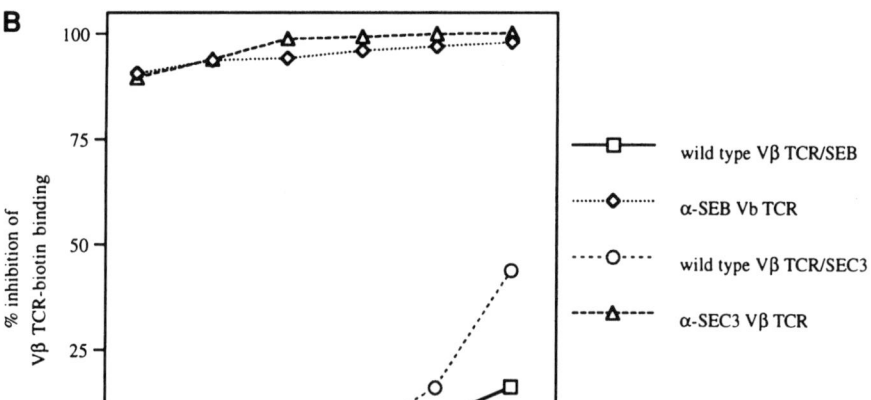

Fig. 2.

monomeric protein can be isolated form 9 L of culture. In contrast to the Trx-αβ TCR, the V_β TCR is present primarily in monomeric form, thus further purification by gel filtration is optional. Up to 6 mg of protein can be isolated form 9 L of culture.

2. If necessary, the Trx-αβ TCR may be concentrated to 1 mg/mL in PBS.
3. Biotinylated wild-type TCR is used at a concentration that yields about 50% maximum signal in a separate titration of biotinylated wild-type TCR on immobilized monoclonal anti-V_β antibodies.
4. $V_\beta 8$-specific competition ELISAs are performed to evaluate the degree of refolding of the TCRs. In order to account for variations in the fraction of properly folded TCR, $V_\beta 8$ reactivity of each TCR is used as a normalization factor in determining SAg reactivity.
5. Biotinylated SAg is used at a concentration that yields about 50% maximum signal in a separate titration of biotinylated SAg on wild-type scTCR.

References

1. Marrack, P. and Kappler, J. (1990) The staphylococcal enterotoxins and their relatives [published erratum appears in Science 1990 Jun 1;248(4959):1066]. *Science* **248,** 705–711.
2. Bentley, G. A., Boulot, G., Karjalainen, K., and Mariuzza, R. A. (1995) Crystal structure of the β chain of a T cell antigen receptor. *Science* **267,** 1984–1987.
3. Fields, B. A., Ober, B., Malchiodi, E. L., Lebedeva, M. I., Braden, B.

Fig. 2. (*see opposite page*) Competition ELISA of TCR mutants with SAgs. (**A**) Inhibition of SEC3-1A4 binding by representative scTCR alanine mutants. Wild-type and mutant scTCRs were used at various concentrations to inhibit the binding of biotinylated SEC3-1A4 to wild-type scTCR in an ELISA format. Bound biotinylated SEC3-1A4 was detected with streptavidin-HRP. The reactivity of each mutant was determined as the ratio of mutant to wild-type IC_{50} by linear regression analysis. (**B**) Relative V_β TCR mutant reactivities for binding SEB and SEC3. Various concentrations of SEB and SEC3 were used to inhibit binding of biotinylated wild-type and mutant V_β TCRs to immobilized anti-$V_\beta 8$ MAb KJ16 in an ELISA format. Bound biotinylated V_β TCR was detected with SAv-HRP.

C., Ysern, X., et al. (1995) Crystal structure of the Vα domain of a T cell antigen receptor. *Science* **270**, 1821–1824.

4. Garcia, K. C., Degano, M., Stanfield, R. L., Brunmark, A., Jackson, M. R., Peterson, P. A., et al. (1996) An αβ T cell receptor structure at 2.5 angstrom and its orientation in the TCR-MHC complex. *Science* **274**, 209–219.

5. Garboczi, D. N., Ghosh, P., Utz, U., Fan, Q. R., Biddison, W. E., and Wiley, D. C. (1996) Structure of the complex between human T-cell receptor, viral peptide and HLA-A2. *Nature* **384**, 131–141.

6. Fields, B. A., Malchiodi, E. L., Li, H., Ysern, X., Stauffacher, C. V., Schlievert, P. M., et al. (1996) Crystal structure of a T-cell receptor β-chain complexed with a superantigen. *Nature* **384**, 188–192.

7. Li, H., Llera, A., Tsuchiya, D., Leder, L., Ysern, X., Schlievert, P. M., et al. (1998) Three-dimensional structure of the complex between a T cell receptor beta chain and the superantigen staphylococcal enterotoxin B. *Immunity* **9**, 807–816.

8. Malchiodi, E. L., Eisenstein, E., Fields, B. A., Ohlendorf, D. H., Schlievert, P. M., Karjalainen, K., and Mariuzza, R. A. (1995) Superantigen binding to a T cell receptor β chain of known three-dimensional structure. *J. Exp. Med.* **182**, 1833–1845.

9. Leder, L., Llera, A., Lavoie, P. M., Lebedeva, M. I., Li, H., Sekaly, R. P., et al. (1998) A mutational analysis of the binding of staphylococcal enterotoxins B and C3 to the T cell receptor beta chain and major histocompatibility complex class II. *J. Exp. Med.* **187**, 823–833.

10. Andersen, P. S., Lavoie, P. M., Sekaly, R. P., Churchill, H., Kranz, D. M., Schlievert, P. M., et al. (1999) Role of the T cell receptor alpha chain in stabilizing TCR-superantigen- MHC class II complexes. *Immunity* **10**, 473–483.

11. Churchill, H. R., Andersen, P. S., Parke, E. A., Mariuzza, R. A., and Kranz, D. M. (2000) Mapping the energy of superantigen Staphylococcus enterotoxin C3 recognition of an alpha/beta T cell receptor using alanine scanning mutagenesis. *J. Exp. Med.* **191**, 835–846.

12. Andersen, P. S., Geisler, C., Buus, S., Mariuzza, R. A., and Karjalainen, K. (2001) Role of TCR-ligand affinity in T cell activation by bacterial superantigens. *J. Biol. Chem.* **276**, 33,452–33,456.

13. Kappler, J., White, J., Kozono, H., Clements, J., and Marrack, P. (1994) Binding of a soluble αβ T-cell receptor to superantigen/major histocompatibility complex ligands. *Proc. Natl. Acad. Sci. USA* **91**, 8462–8466.

14. Khandekar, S. S., Brauer, P. P., Naylor, J. W., Chang, H. C., Kern, P., Newcomb, J. R., et al. (1997) Affinity and kinetics of the interactions between an alphabeta T-cell receptor and its superantigen and class II-MHC/peptide ligands. *Mol. Immunol.* **34,** 493–503.

15. Schodin, B. A., Schlueter, C. J., and Kranz, D. M. (1996) Binding properties and solubility of single-chain T cell receptors expressed in *E. coli. Mol. Immunol.* **33,** 819–829.

16. Kieke, M. C., Sundberg, E., Shusta, E. V., Mariuzza, R. A., Wittrup, K. D., and Kranz, D. M. (2001) High affinity T cell receptors from yeast display libraries block T cell activation by superantigens. *J. Mol. Biol.* **307,** 1305–1315.

17. Kranz, D. M., Sherman, D. H., Sitkovsky, M. V., Pasternack, M. S., and Eisen, H. N. (1984) Immunoprecipitation of cell surface structure of cloned cytotoxic T lymphocytes by clone-specific antisera. Proc. Natl. Acad. Sci. USA **81,** 573–577.

18. Soo Hoo, W. F., Lacy, M. J., Denzin, L. K., Voss, E. W. J., Hardman, K. D., and Kranz, D. M. (1992) Characterization of a single-chain T cell receptor expressed in *E. coli. Proc. Natl. Acad. Sci. USA* **89,** 4759–4763.

19. Haskins, K., Hannum, C., White, J., Rhoem, N., Kubo, R., Kappler, J., and Marrack, K. (1984) The antigen-specific major histocompatibility complex-restricted receptor on T cells. VI. An antibody to a receptor allotype. *J. Exp. Med.* **160,** 452–471.

20. Staerz, U. D., Rammensee, H. G., Benedetto, J. D., and Bevan, M. J. (1985) Characterization of a murine monoclonal antibody specific for an allotypic determinant on T cell antigen receptor. *J. Immunol.* **134,** 3994–4000.

8

Role of Accessory Molecules in the Superantigen-Induced Activation of Peripheral Blood T Cells

Catherine Gelin, Marie-Thérèse Zilber,
and Dominique Charron

1. Introduction

Among the antigens presented by the major histocompatibility complex (MHC) class II molecules, the superantigens (SAgs) constitute a particular family of ligands that are able to signal via the MHC class II molecules *(1)*. The SAg are characterized by their ability to bind to both the MHC class II molecules *(2,3)* and to the V_β region of the TCR *(4)*. The formation of this trimolecular complex results in the activation of all T cells bearing the appropriate T-cell receptor (TCR) V_β family *(5)*. This T-cell activation by SAg has been described as being MHC class II molecule-dependent (although unrestricted). However, the expression of MHC class II molecules on some antigen-presenting cells (APCs) is not always sufficient to induce a T-cell response to the SAg as was observed in studies of MHC class II expressing astrocytes *(6)*, keratinocytes *(7)* and a class II-transfected L line *(8)*. These results could be interpreted as suggesting that co-stimulatory molecules are necessary, in addition to MHC class II molecules, to lead to a full response to SAg.

From: *Methods in Molecular Biology, vol. 214: Superantigen Protocols*
Edited by: T. Krakauer © Humana Press Inc., Totowa, NJ

The starting point of our studies was the search of the co-accessory molecules necessary on APC, to implement a valid signal during T-cell activation by SAg. The basic idea was to use monoclonal antibodies (Mabs) specific for surface molecules expressed on accessory cells and to evaluate the influence of the subsequent ligation on a SAg-induced T cell proliferation. We have thus described the role of CD1a *(9,10)* and CD38 *(11)* molecules as co-accessory molecules of the SAg-induced responses.

We will describe some of the techniques that have allowed us to obtain the results leading to these conclusions. We will review the techniques used to obtain purified T cells and monocytes preparations, and the proliferation assay.

2. Materials

1. Peripheral blood cells prepared by Ficoll-Paque density centrifugation of buffy coats obtained from the local blood bank.
2. Ficoll-Paque (Pharmacia, Uppsala, Sweden).
3. Complement-fixing MAbs (anti-MHC class II, CD3).
4. RPMI 1640 medium (Biochrom KG, Berlin, Germany) supplemented with 2 mM L-glutamine, 10 U/mL penicillin, 10 µg/mL streptomycin (Gibco, Paisley, UK).
5. Normal human serum (previously decomplemented for 1 h at 56°C, aliquoted, and stored at –20°C).
6. Fetal calf serum (previously decomplemented for 1 h at 56°C, aliquoted, and stored at –20°C) (Seromed, Biochrom KG, Berlin, Germany).
7. RPMI medium containing 20% normal human serum (RPMI-20% NHS).
8. RPMI medium containing 10% fetal calf serum (RPMI-10% FCS).
9. Rabbit serum complement (aliquoted, stored at –80°C and diluted just before use) (Filorga, Paris, France).
10. 15- and 50-mL polypropylene tubes (Falcon).
11. 75 cm^2 culture flasks (Falcon).
12. 96-well round-bottom microtiter plates with lids (Nunc).
13. Purified MAbs (CD3, CD19, CD14, anti-MHC class II, and MAbs

which will be tested for their influence in SAg-induced proliferation) either locally produced or purchased from Coulter/Immunotech (Marseille, France).

14. Phosphate-buffered saline (PBS).
15. Paraformaldehyde.
16. (^{3}H) thymidine (Amersham, Little Chalfont, UK).
17. Purified or recombinant superantigen (TSST-1 or SEA) (Sigma, Saint-Quentin Fallavier, France).
18. Phytohemagglutinin (PHA) (Difco, Detroit, MI).

3. Methods

3.1. T-Cell Enrichment

Purified T cells are obtained by the following negative selection procedure: two cycles of plastic adherence and one cycle of complement-dependent lysis. T cells from peripheral blood do not express the MHC class II molecules. This characteristic is used to enrich for T cells, obtained after plastic adherence, using cytotoxic anti-MHC class II MAb and activating complement. Lymphocyte suspensions are incubated with an MHC class II MAb first. Complement previously screened for low toxicity is then added to lyse the cells labeled with the anti-MHC class II MAb.

3.1.1. T-Cell Enrichment by Plastic Adherence

This step uses the ability of accessory cells, monocytes, to adhere to plastic of culture flasks and thus lead to a population enriched in T cells in the nonadherent fraction.

1. Peripheral blood cells prepared by Ficoll-Paque density centrifugation are resuspended in RPMI-20% NHS (1×10^6 cells/mL).
2. Cell suspension is aliquoted in 75 cm^2 culture flasks (20 mL/flask). Flasks are then stored horizontally for 1 h in a humidified 37°C, 5% CO$_2$ incubator.
3. Nonadherent cells are removed, and subjected to a second cycle of adherence on new flasks for 1 h at 37°C. Nonadherent cells obtained from the two cycles of plastic adherence are washed twice in RPMI. These nonadherent cells are enriched in T cells.

3.1.2. T-Cell Purification by Cytotoxic Elimination of B and Accessory Cells

This step will eliminate B and accessory cells that have not adhered to plastic and thus contaminated the T-cell preparation.

1. In 50 mL polypropylene tubes, enriched T-cell population (40×10^6 cells) is resuspended in 2 mL cytotoxic anti-MHC class II MAb diluted in RPMI (final dilution ~1–5 µg/mL) (*see* **Note 1**), and incubated 20 min at 4°C.
2. Rabbit serum complement is added at the dilution established for low toxicity and high specificity (final dilution ~ 1:4 to 1:10) (*see* **Note 2**), and the cell suspension is incubated for 45 min at 37°C.
3. Cells are then washed three times in RPMI by centrifugation at 200g for 10 min.
4. Pellets are resuspended in RPMI for viability test with trypan blue, flow cytometer analysis, and functional assays (*see* **Notes 3** and **4**).

3.2. Monocyte Enrichment

Purified monocytes are obtained by the following negative selection procedure: two cycles of plastic adherence and one cycle of complement-dependent lysis. Monocytes do not express the CD3 molecules. This characteristic is used to enrich for monocytes, obtained after plastic adherence, using cytotoxic CD3 MAb and activating complement.

1. Peripheral blood cells were resuspended in RPMI-20% NHS (1×10^6 cells/mL).
2. Cell suspension is aliquoted in 75 cm^2 culture flasks (20 mL/flask). Flasks are then stored horizontally for 1 h in a humidified 37°C, 5% CO_2 incubator.
3. Nonadherent cells are removed, and subjected to a second cycle of adherence on new flasks for 1 h at 37°C.
4. Adherent cells obtained from the two cycles of adherence are collected immediately after incubation at 37°C by adding 5 mL of cold RPMI to the flask, and scrapping the flask with a rubber policeman. Adherent cells are collected in a 50-mL tube.
5. Adherent cells are further subjected to T cell depletion by cytotoxic elimination as described in the unit "T-cell enrichment." However,

CD3-specific MAb is used (rather than MHC class II MAb) to eliminate T cells (rather than MHC class II positive cells) (*see* **Notes 5** and **6**).

3.3. Monocyte Fixation

In some experiments fixed monocytes precoated with specific
MAbs are used to evaluate the role of the recognized molecules in
the superantigen-induced proliferation

1. Pellets of adherent cells (20×10^6 cells),obtained from the above
   techniques, are resuspended either in 2 mL of purified MAbs
   (~5–10 μg/mL) diluted in RPMI (precoated-fixed monocytes) or in
   2 mL RPMI (fixed monocytes) and incubated for 1 h at 4°C.
2. Cells are washed twice in RPMI.
3. Pellets are resuspended in PBS buffer containing 1% paraformaldehyde, and incubated for 25 min at room temperature.
4. Cells are washed three times in RMPI resuspended at 2×10^5 cells/mL
   and kept at 4°C in RPMI-10% FCS, at least 3 wk before use (*see*
   Note 7).

3.4. Superantigen-Induced T-Cell Proliferation

To evaluate the influence of different monocyte surface molecules in a superantigen-induced activation, a proliferative assay
induced by superantigens with peripheral blood cells in the presence of monoclonal antibodies specific for the molecules is studied
first (*see* **Fig. 1**) *(9)*. To assess the specific role of the monocyte
surface molecule, a second proliferative assay is performed with
purified T cells and MAb-precoated fixed monocytes.

3.4.1. Proliferation Assay with Peripheral Blood Cells

1. Peripheral blood cell suspension prepared by Ficoll-Paque density centrifugation are resuspended in RPMI-10% FCS at 1×10^6 cells /mL.
   For the standard protocol described in **Table 1**, 5 mL of peripheral
   blood cells at 1×10^6 cells/mL should be prepared for each plate.
2. A series of four dilutions of MAbs, including isotype control MAbs
   as negative controls, are prepared in RPMI-10% FCS: 3, 7.5, 15, and
   30 μg/mL. These dilutions will lead to a final concentration of MAb

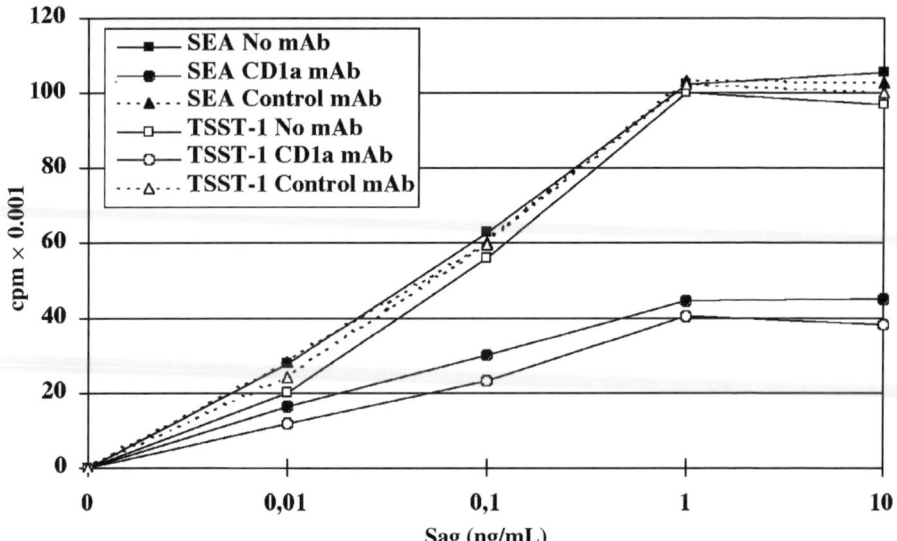

Fig. 1. The proliferative response of CD1(+) peripheral blood cells to SEA and TSST-1 is inhibited by CD1a MAbs. CD1(+) Peripheral blood cells (5×10^4 cells/well) were cultured with varied concentrations of SEA or TSST-1 in the presence of CD1a MAb L544 or isotype control CD99 (5 µg/mL). Cultures were pulsed after 90 h with 1 µCi/well ^{3}H-thymidine, then harvested for scintillation counting at d 4. The results of one experiment, representative of five, are expressed as mean counts per minute of triplicate determinations. SDs were typically <15%.

in the well of 1, 2.5, 5, and 10 µg/mL respectively. For a standard protocol described in **Table 1**, 600 µL of each dilution will be necessary, but to avoid problems during redistribution in wells, 700 µL should be prepared.

3. A series of 4 dilutions of SAg are prepared in RPMI-10% FCS: 0.3, 3, 30, and 300 ng/mL). These dilutions will lead to a final concentration of SAg in the well of 0.1, 1, 10, and 100 ng/mL respectively. For a standard protocol described in **Table 1**, 900 µL of each dilution will be necessary, but to avoid problems during redistribution in wells, 1 mL should be prepared.

4. PHA, used as a positive control of proliferation, is diluted in RPMI-10% FCS at 150 ng/mL final.

5. 50 μL of peripheral blood cell suspension are added to each well of a 96-well round-bottom microtiter plate. Each well of the plate will thus contain 5×10^4 cells.
6. Microtiter plates can be organized as indicated in **Table 1**. 50 μL of diluted MAbs are added to the cells. A series of four dilution for each MAb will form one row of each plate. A control of three wells with 50 μL of RPMI-10% FCS in the place of MAb should be included.
7. The plates are placed at room temperature for 30 min to allow binding of MAbs.
8. 50 μL of diluted SAg, PHA, or RPMI-10% FCS are added to the cells as indicated in **Table 1**.
9. Microtiter plates are placed in a humidified 37°C, 5% CO_2 incubator for 4 d.
10. 1 μCi of (^{3}H)thymidine (5Ci/mM) is added to each well for the last 8 h of culture.
11. At the end of d 4, plates are harvested with a TOMTEC harvester (TOMTEC, CA) and the radioactivity is measured in a β scintillation counter (1450 Microbeta Plus, Wallac, Finland).

The dilutions of MAbs and SAg determined in these conditions will be used next for further proliferation studies.

3.4.2. Proliferation Assay with Purified T-Cells and Fixed Autologous Monocytes

SAg induce a strong T-cell proliferative response. This stimulation requires binding of SAg to the V_β region of the TCR. Using purified T cells from peripheral blood cells, no proliferative response will be induced in the absence of accessory cells, as this response also requires SAg fixation to the MHC class II molecules. To restore T-cell response to SAg, irradiated or paraformaldehyde fixed autologous monocytes should be added (*see* **Table 2**) (*9*).

1. Purified T-cell suspension prepared as described earlier are resuspended in RPMI-10% FCS at 1×10^6 cells /mL. For the standard protocol described in **Table 2**, 1.5 mL of purified T cells at 1×10^6 cells/mL should be prepared for each plate
2. For the standard protocol described in **Table 3**, 1 mL of fixed monocytes and 200 μL of each precoated fixed autologous monocytes,

Table 1
Organization of Microtiter Plates for SAg-Induced Proliferation Assays with Peripheral Blood Cells

Row	Wells 1–3[a]	Wells 4–6	Wells 7–9	Well 10–12
Lane 1	Medium (100 μL/well)	PHA (100 μL/well)		
Lane 2	SAg dilution 1 (50 μL/well) Medium (50 μL/well)	SAg dilution 2 (50 μL/well) Medium (50 μL/well)	SAg dilution 3 (50 μL/well) Medium (50 μL/well)	SAg dilution 4 (50 μL/well) Medium (50 μL/well)
Lane 3[b]	SAg dilution 1 (50 μL/well) MAb1 dilution 1 (50 μL/well)	SAg dilution 1 (50 μL/well) MAb1 dilution 2 (50 μL/well)	SAg dilution 1 (50 μL/well) MAb1 dilution 3 (50 μL/well)	SAg dilution 1 (50 μL/well) MAb1 dilution 4 (50 μL/well)
Lane 4	SAg dilution 2 (50 μL/well) MAb1 dilution 1 (50 μL/well)	SAg dilution 2 (50 μL/well) MAb1 dilution 2 (50 μL/well)	SAg dilution 2 (50 μL/well) MAb1 dilution 3 (50 μL/well)	SAg dilution 2 (50 μL/well) MAb1 dilution 4 (50 μL/well)
Lane 5	SAg dilution 3 (50 μL/well) MAb1 dilution 1 (50 μL/well)	SAg dilution 3 (50 μL/well) MAb1 dilution 2 (50 μL/well)	SAg dilution 3 (50 μL/well) MAb1 dilution 3 (50 μL/well)	SAg dilution 3 (50 μL/well) MAb1 dilution 4 (50 μL/well)
Lane 6	SAg dilution 4 (50 μL/well) MAb1 dilution 1 (50 μL/well)	SAg dilution 4 (50 μL/well) MAb1 dilution 2 (50 μL/well)	SAg dilution 4 (50 μL/well) MAb1 dilution 3 (50 μL/well)	SAg dilution 4 (50 μL/well) MAb1 dilution 4 (50 μL/well)
Lane 7	SAg dilution 1 (50 μL/well) control MAb (50 μL/well)	SAg dilution 2 (50 μL/well) control MAb (50 μL/well)	SAg dilution 3 (50 μL/well) control MAb (50 μL/well)	SAg dilution 4 (50 μL/well) control MAb (50 μL/well)
Lane 8				

[a]Each well contains 50 μL of cell suspension at 1×10^6 cells/mL.
[b]Lane 3–7 are repeated for each MAb tested.

Table 2
Role of the Monocyte Surface CD1a Molecule in SAg-Induced Proliferation of T Cells

Purified T cells incubated with[a]	SEA	% Inh[b]	TSST-1	% Inh
Medium	0.6 ± 0.2	—	0.3 ± 0.1	—
fM	30.0 ± 0.2	—	25.0 ± 1.3	—
fM + soluble CD1a MAb L544	13.5 ± 0.5	(55%)	10.0 ± 0.6	(60%)
fM + soluble CD1a MAb UN5	12.9 ± 1.0	(57%)	10.5 ± 0.7	(58%)
fM + soluble MHC class II MAb	9.1 ± 0.5	(69%)	7.5 ± 0.8	(70%)
fM precoated with CD1a MAb L544	12.0 ± 0.8	(60%)	9.2 ± 0.8	(64%)
fM precoated with CD1a MAb UN5	12.3 ± 0.5	(59%)	8.7 ± 0.5	(65%)
fM precoated with CD1b MAb O249	28.1 ± 1.0	(06%)	24.1 ± 0.5	(04%)
fM precoated with CD1c MAb L161	29.3 ± 0.9	(03%)	25.0 ± 0.7	(00%)
fM precoated with MHC Class II MAb	7.5 ± 0.8	(75%)	8.0 ± 0.5	(68%)
fM precoated with control MAb	28.7 ± 0.8	(04%)	23.2 ± 1.0	(07%)

[a]Whole purified T cells (4×10^4 cells/well) were cultured either alone or with fixed monocytes (fM) (8×10^3 cells/well) with or without MAb of the indicated specificity (5 μg/mL). T-cell proliferation induced by SEA or TSST-1 (both at 1 ng/mL) was measured at d 4.
[b]Percent inhibition of the T-cell proliferation.

Table 3
Organization of Microtiter Plates for SAg-Induced Proliferation Assays with Purified T-Cells and Fixed Monocytes

Row	Wells 1–3	Wells 4–6	Wells 7–9	Wells 10–12
Lane 1	T cells (40 µL/well)	T cells (40 µL/well)	fM (40 µL/well)	fM (40 µL/well)
		PHA (40 µL/well)		PHA (40 µL/well)
	Medium (120 µL/well)	Medium (80 µL/well)	Medium (120 µL/well)	Medium (80 µL/w(
Lane 2	T cells (40 µL/well)	fM (40 µL/well)	T cells (40 µL/well)	T cells (40 µL/we
			fM (40 µL/well)	fM (40 µL/well)
	SAg (40 µL/well)	SAg (40 µL/well)	PHA (40 µL/well)	SAg (40 µL/well)
	Medium (80 µL/well)	Medium (80 µL/well)	Medium (40 µL/well)	Medium (40 µL/w(
Lane 3	T cells (40 µL/well)	T cells (40 µL/well)	T cells (40 µL/well)	
	fM (40 µL/well)	fM (40 µL/well)	fM (40 µL/well)	
	MAb1(40 µL/well)	Class II MAb (40 µL/well)	control MAb (40 µL/well)	
	SAg (40 µL/well)	SAg (40 µL/well)	SAg (40 µL/well)	
Lane 4	T cells (40 µL/well)	T cells (40 µL/well)	T cells (40 µL/well)	
	MAb-fM (40 µL/well)	class II MAb-fM (40 µL/well)	control MAb-fM (40 µL/well)	
	SAg (40 µL/well)	SAg (40 µL/well)	SAg (40 µL/well)	
	Medium (40 µL/well)	Medium (40 µL/well)	Medium (40 µL/well)	
Lane 5				
Lane 6				
Lane 7				
Lane 8				

122

prepared according to the protocol described earlier, are washed twice in RPMI-10%FCS and resuspended without counting in the initial volume of RPMI-10% FCS.

3. The MAbs are diluted in RPMI-10% FCS at the dilution established from the above protocol. For the standard protocol described in **Table 3**, 150 μL of diluted MAb should be prepared.

4. The SAg is diluted in RPMI-10% FCS at the dilution established from the aforementioned protocol. For the standard protocol described in **Table 3**, 1.2 mL of diluted SAg should be prepared.

5. PHA, used as a positive control of proliferation, is diluted in RMPI-10% FCS at 150 ng/mL final.

6. Microtiter plates can be organized as indicated in **Table 3**. 40 μL of purified T cells are added to each of indicated well of a 96-well round-bottom microtiter plate. Each indicated well of the plate will thus contain 4×10^4 cells.

7. 40 μL of fixed or precoated fixed monocytes are added to each indicated well. Each indicated well will thus contain 8×10^3 cells.

8. 40 μL of diluted MAb are added to each indicated well.

9. The plates are placed at room temperature for 30 min to allow binding of MAbs.

10. 50 μL of diluted SAg, PHA, or RPMI-10% FCS are added to the cells as indicated in **Table 3**.

11. Microtiter plates are placed in a humidified 37°C, 5% CO_2 incubator for 4 d.

12. 1 μCi of [^{3}H]thymidine (5 Ci/mM) is added to each well for the last 8 h of culture.

13. At the end of d 4, plates are harvested with a TOMTEC harvester (TOMTEC, CA) and the radioactivity is measured in a β scintillation counter (1450 Microbeta Plus).

3.4.3. Analysis of the Results of Proliferative Responses

1. The median value of each triplicate is calculated (*see* **Note 8**).

2. Median cpm of controls containing peripheral blood cells or purified T cells in the absence of stimulation should be <1000 cpm (*see* **Note 9**).

3. The proliferative results are calculated by the difference in median cpm of stimulated (in the presence of SAg) cells and control (without SAg) cells.

4. Median cpm of the proliferative response of fresh peripheral blood cells induced by the toxins SEA or TSST-1 should be around 100,000 cpm, while the response observed with purified T cells and fixed autologous monocytes will reach a maximum of around 40,000 cpm (*see* **Note 10**).

5. To evaluate the influence of a surface molecule ligation with a specific MAb on the SAg-induced proliferative response, percent inhibition of the proliferative response is calculated as follow: $100 \times$ [(median cpm of proliferation in the absence of MAb) – (median cpm of proliferation in the presence of MAb)] / [(median cpm of proliferation in the absence of MAb)].

4. Notes

1. Cytotoxic elimination of accessory cells with anti-MHC class II MAb or of T cells with CD3 MAb does not require the use of purified MAbs. Supernatant or ascitis can be used successfully.

2. The success of cytotoxic elimination depends on critical preliminary tests to establish adequate dilutions of complement. These tests can be performed as follow: tube no.1 with cells and cytoxic MAb (negative control of lysis), tube nos. 2–6 with cells and different dilutions of complement, ranging from 1:4–1:10 (control of complement toxicity), tube nos. 7–10 with cells, MAb, and different dilutions of complement (test of the specificity of lysis)

3. To evaluate their purity, purified T cells obtained are first phenotypically tested by labeling with MAbs specific for T cells, B cells, and monocytes and analyzing by flow cytometry. A typical phenotype of the purified T cells obtained by this negative selection procedure is: >97% of $CD3^+$ cells, <1% of $CD19^+$ cells, <1% of $CD14^+$ cells, and <1% of MHC class II+ cells. As these cells will be used in proliferation assays, another criterion of their purity is their inability to proliferate under PHA stimulation without addition of accessory cells. Such a control must be added in all proliferation assays using purified T cells.

4. Purified T cells will be used in SAg-induced assays with fixed monocytes. For this, the purified T cells should be frozen to allow the time for preparation of fixed monocytes, which should be kept at 4°C for several weeks before use (*see* **Note 7**)

5. To evaluate their purity, purified monocytes obtained are phenotypically tested by labeling with MAbs specific for T cells, B cells, and

monocytes and analyzed by flow cytometry. A typical phenotype of the purified monocytes obtained by this negative selection procedure is: <1% of CD3$^+$ cells, >98% of CD14$^+$ cells, and >98% of MHC class II+ cells.

6. While we have described separately the procedures leading to T-cell enrichment and to monocyte enrichment, in practice these procedures are concomitant: peripheral blood cells are subjected to plastic adherence as described and the adherent cells or nonadherent cells are collected, subjected to cytotoxic elimination with CD3 or MHC class II Mabs, respectively, leading to purified monocytes or purified T cells, respectively. One day should be sufficient for obtaining peripheral blood cells from blood samples, adherence procedures, cytotoxic elimination, washes, and counting. The purified cells can be stored at 4°C overnight in RPMI-10% FCS before phenotypic analysis by flow cytometry.

7. Fixed monocytes should be kept at least 3 wk at 4°C and washed extensively before use to avoid toxicity due to paraformaldehyde. In fact the older the fixed monocytes, the better they will perform in proliferation assays. The concentration of these fixed monocytes is adjusted at 2×10^5 cells/mL at the end of the procedure and will be used at this concentration without further counting.

8. Technical problems related to errors in dilutions or pipetting can lead to aberrant triplicate values. In this case the aberrant values are omitted in the results.

9. If bacterial contaminations occur during the cell culture, a strong [^{3}H] thymidine incorporation will be observed in the controls containing peripheral blood cells or purified T cells in the absence of stimulation, and the results obtained in such experiments should not be considered.

10. Very efficient proliferative responses are observed with fresh cells. However, the proliferative assays can be performed with frozen peripheral blood cells leading to slightly lowest responses (~50,000 cpm). Cells are frozen in FCS containing 10% DMSO in liquid nitrogen.

References

1. Marrack, P. and Kappler, J. (1994) The staphylococcal enterotoxins and their relatives. *Science* **248,** 705–711.

2. Jardetzky, T. S., Brown, J. H., Gorga, J. C., Stern, J. L., Urban, R. G., Chi, Y., et al. (1994) Three dimensional structure of a human class II histocompatibility molecule complexed with superantigen. *Nature* **368,** 711–718.

3. Seth, A., Stern, L. J., Ottenhoff, T. H., Engel, I., Owen, M. J., Lamb, J. R., et al. (1994) Binary and ternary complexes between T-cell receptor, class II MHC and superantigen in vitro. *Nature* **369,** 324–327.

4. Kappler, J., Kotzin, B., Herron, L., Gelfand, E. W., Bigler, R. D., Boylston, A., et al. (1989) V_β-specific stimulation of human T cells by staphylococcal toxins. *Science* **244,** 811–813.

5. Webb, S. R. and Gascoigne, N. R. (1994) T cell activation by superantigens. *Curr. Opin. Immunol.* **6,** 467–475.

6. Rott, O., Tontsh, U., and Fleischer, B. (1993) Dissociation of antigen-presenting capacity of astrocytes for peptide-antigen versus superantigen . *J. Immunol.* **150,** 87–95.

7. Nickoloff, B. J., Mitra, R. S., Green, J., Zheng, X. G., Shimizu, Y., Thompson, C., and Turka, L. A. (1993) Accessory cell function of keratinocytes for superantigens. Dependence on LFA-1/ICAM-1 interaction. *J. Immunol.* **150,** 2148–2159.

8. Yagi, J., Uchiyama, U., and Janeway, C. A. (1994) Stimulator cell type influences the response of T cells to staphylococcal enterotoxins. *J. Immunol.* **152,** 1154–1162.

9. Gregory, S., Zilber, M-T., Charron, D., and Gelin, C. (2000) Human CD1a molecule expressed on monocytes plays an accessory role in the superantigen-induced activation of T lymphocytes. *Human Immunol.* **61,** 193–201.

10. Gregory, S., Zilber, M.-T., Choqueux, C., Mooney, N., Charron, D., and Gelin, C. (2000) Role of the CD1a molecule in the superantigen induced activation of MHC class II negative thymocytes. *Human Immunol.* **61,** 427–437.

11. Zilber, M.-T., Gregory, S., Mallone, R., Deaglio, S., Malavasi, F., Charron, D., and Gelin, C. (2000) CD38 expressed on human monocytes: a co-accessory molecule in the superantigen-induced proliferation. *Proc. Natl. Acad. Sci. USA* **97,** 2840–2845.

9

T-Lymphocyte Activation Induced by Staphylococcal Enterotoxin Superantigens

Analysis of Protein Tyrosine Phosphorylation

Anne Roumier, Florence Niedergang, and Andrés Alcover

1. Introduction

Staphylococcus enterotoxin superantigens (SAgs) have the capacity to strongly activate oligoclonal populations of T lymphocytes expressing T-cell antigen receptors (TCR) that share particular V_β elements. These superantigens stimulate T lymphocytes by binding simultaneously to TCR V_β domains and to major histocompatibility complex (MHC) class II molecules on antigen-presenting cells (APCs) *(1)*. Several characteristics distinguish enterotoxin superantigens from conventional antigens: (1) superantigen stimulation, although usually requiring the presence of MHC class II molecules on APCs, is not restricted to one MHC allele. Therefore, *a priori* any MHC class II positive cell would be suitable as superantigen presenting cell. (2) Processing of superantigens into antigenic peptides is not necessary. Therefore, just short incubations are necessary to pulse APCs with enterotoxin superantigens.

From: *Methods in Molecular Biology, vol. 214: Superantigen Protocols*
Edited by: T. Krakauer © Humana Press Inc., Totowa, NJ

Here we describe the use of enterotoxin superantigens as T-cell stimulators to analyze tyrosine-phosphorylated associated with the TCR-CD3 complex or from total cell lysates, as used for instance in *(2)*. The involvement of protein tyrosine kinases in the TCR signaling cascade has been extensively studied (reviewed in **refs.** *[3, 4]*). However, it is important to keep in mind that qualitative or quantitative differences in tyrosine-phosphorylated polypeptides are often found in the literature. These differences may be owing to the cellular systems studied (i.e., peripheral blood T-cells, lectin-activated T-cell blasts, T-cell clones, tumor Jurkat T cells, T-cell hybridomas, splenic T cells, etc.), to the kind of stimulus used to activate the T cells (i.e., peptide antigen, enterotoxin superantigens, anti-TCR or anti-CD3 monoclonal antibodies, [MAbs] etc.), or to the quality of the stimulus (i.e., antibodies of different isotypes, enterotoxin superantigens displaying different affinities for the different T-cell receptors, the type of APCs, etc.) Enterotoxin superantigens are in most cases very efficient T-cell activators, when compared with antigenic peptides, or with anti-TCR-CD3 MAbs, inducing stronger and longer-lasting protein tyrosine phosphorylation (*see* **Fig. 1**).

2. Materials

2.1. Buffers and Solutions

1. Enterotoxin stock solutions are made at 1 mg/mL in sterile phosphate-buffered saline (PBS), alliquoted and kept frozen at –20°C. Once thawed, the solutions were kept at 4°C.
2. Sodium orthovanadate (10 mM stock solution). Weight the Na_3VO_4 and dissolve it in 45 mL of distilled water. Measure the pH (it will be around 11.5), and adjust it to pH 10.0 using 1 M HCl. The solution turns into yellow color. Boil the solution until it becomes clear. Measure again the pH (it will be around 7.5–8.0). Adjust the pH to 10.0 using 1 M NaOH. Add distilled water to 50 mL. Filter and keep at room temperature.
3. Lysis buffer: 20 mM Tris-HCl, pH 7.5, 150 mM NaCl, 1% Brij 97 detergent is kept at 4°C. Just before use, the following phosphatase

total lysates

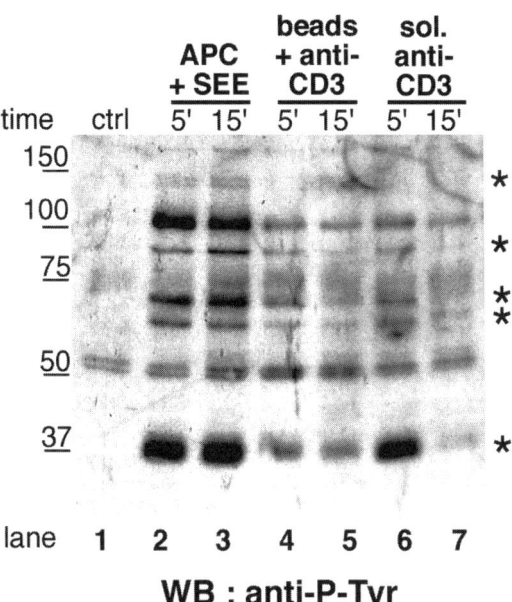

WB : anti-P-Tyr

Fig. 1. Pattern of tyrosine phosphorylated proteins in total cell extracts from cells activated with enterotoxin superantigen or with anti-CD3 MAb. Jurkat T cells were activated with SEE superantigen (lanes 1–3), or with anti-CD3 MAb (UCHT-1), either coupled to sepharose beads to better cross-link TCR-CD3 complexes (lanes 4–6), or in soluble form (lanes 5–7). Six major tyrosine phosphorylated polypeptides were detected (positions marked by stars on the right side). Of note is that tyrosine phosphorylation of proteins from SEE-activated cells appeared more intense and lasted for longer time than those from cells activated with anti-CD3 Ab.

and protease inhibitors are added at the following final concentrations: 1 mM EGTA, 50 mM NaF, 1 mM NaVO4, 10 μg/mL leupeptin, 10 μg/mL aprotinin, 1 mM phenylmethylsulfonyl fluoride (PMSF) (*see* **Note 1**).

4. Immunoprecipitation washing buffer: 20 mM Tris-HCl, pH 7.5, 150 mM NaCl, 1% Brij 97.
5. Transfer buffer: 25 mM Tris-base, 190 mM glycine, 20% ethanol (*see* **Note 2**).

6. Ponceau S solution for membrane staining: 0.2% Ponceau S, 5% trichloroacetic acid (TCA) in distilled water.
7. PBS: 10 mM phosphate buffer, pH 7.4, 137 mM NaCl, 5 mM KCl.
8. Western blotting membrane blocking buffer: 0.1% Tween-20, 1% gelatin in PBS.
9. Western blotting Ab incubation buffer: 0.1% Tween-20, 0.1% gelatin in PBS.
10. Western blotting wash buffer: 0.1% Tween-20 in PBS.

2.2. Reagents

1. *Staphylococcus aureus* enterotoxin (SE) superantigens (Toxin Technology, Madison, WI).
2. Anti-CD3 MAb OKT3 (IgG2a) (American Type Culture Collection [ATCC], Rockville, MD).
3. Anti-phosphotyrosine MAb, 4G10 (Upstate Biotechnology Inc., Lake Placid, NY).
4. Horseradish peroxidase-linked anti-mouse Ig Abs (Amersham-Pharmacia Biotech).
5. Enhance chemiluminiscence (ECL) Western blotting reagents (Amersham-Pharmacia Biotech).
6. Protein A-Sepharose (Amersham-Phamacia Biotech).
7. Brij-97 detergent (polyoxyethylene 10 oleyl ether) (Sigma, St Louis, MO).
8. Tween-20 (polyoxyethylene-sorbitan monolaurate) detergent (Sigma).
9. Cell-culture media and reagents (Gibco-BRL, Rockville, MD).
10. Polyacrylamide gel elecrophoresis (PAGE) solutions (Bio-Rad, Hercules, CA).
11. Ponceau-S (Serva, Heidelberg, Germany).

2.3. Cells

1. The human leukemia T-cell line Jurkat is available from the ATCC.
2. The Burkitt B-cell lymphoma Raji (used here as APCs) is available from the ATCC.

Cell lines are cultured in RPMI-1640, supplemented with 10% fetal calf serum (FCS) and 10 mM HEPES buffer, pH 7.3. Cells are used when growing exponentially, usually between $2–8 \times 10^5$ cells/mL.

2.4. Utilities and Special Equipment

1. Polyvinylidene fluoride (PVDF) membrane (Millipore Corp. Bedford, MA).
2. Liquid protein transfer apparatus, Transblot Cell (Bio-Rad).

3. Methods
3.1. T-Cell Activation

1. Take 10^7 cells per immunoprecipitate of both Jurkat and Raji and resuspend them separately at 2×10^8 cells/mL in serum-free RPMI-1640 medium, supplemented with 10 m*M* HEPES buffer, pH 7.2 (*see* **Note 3**).
2. Split Raji cells into two. To one half, add *Staphylococcus* enterotoxin E (SEE) at 10 µg/mL and incubate them for 15 min at 37°C, in order to pulse the cells with the superantigen.
3. Split Jurkat cells (50 µL per immunoprecipitate) into 1.5-mL conical Eppendorf tubes.
4. Add 50 µL of Raji cell suspension either control or pulsed with SEE superantigen onto the Jurkat cell suspensions. Incubate at 37°C for various times: typically from 1–20 min. (*see* **Notes 4** and **5**).
5. Finish the activation by centrifuging the cell suspension for 10 s at 13,000*g* in a bench-top centrifuge, rapidly remove the supernatant.

3.2. Cell Lysis

1. Add 100 µL of ice-cold lysis buffer per tube containing 10^7 cells, and resuspend the cell pellet by vortexing or pipetting. Allow cell lysis to proceed for 15–30 min on ice, vortexing every 5 min.
2. Centrifuge the cells in Eppendorf conical tubes for 15 min at 13,000*g* in a refrigerated centrifuge. This step eliminates nuclei, membrane debris, and insoluble cytoskeleton (*see* **Note 6**).
3. Take out the supernatant for immunoprecipitation or total cell-extract analysis.

3.3. Total Cell-Extract Analysis

1. Take out 5 µL out of the 100 µL of total cell lysate of Jurkat cells or 10–25 µL for peripheral blood T cells.
2. Add distilled water, and SDS-PAGE sample buffer to 100 µL.

3. Use 30 µL to load on a gel for SDS-PAGE. The rest can be kept frozen at –20°C.

3.4. Immunoprecipitation

1. Pre-clearing. Add 1 µg of irrelevant Ab, (or 1 µL of ascites) (*see* **Note 7**) to the lysis supernatant. Incubate for 15 min at 4°C on a rotating wheel. Then, add 20 µL of a 1:1 suspension of protein-A Sepharose beads, and continue the incubation rotating for 1 h at 4°C. Centrifuge the beads for 15 s at 13,000*g* in a bench-top centrifuge, take out the supernatant and repeat the preclearing once more.

2. Specific immunoprecipitation. To the precleared lysis supernatant, add 1 µg (or 1 µL of ascites) of the appropriate Ab. For example, anti-CD3 MAb OKT3, to immunoprecipitate proteins associated to the TCR-CD3 complex. Incubate, rotating for 15 min at 4°C. Then add 10 µL of protein-A sepharose bead suspension (*see* **Note 8**). Incubate rotating for 3–4 h at 4°C. Finally, centrifuge 15 s at 13,000*g*.

3. Remove carefully the supernatant. Wash 4× the beads with 1 mL each of immunoprecipitation washing buffer and once more with PBS without detergent. Leave about 20 µL of volume. Add SDS-PAGE sample buffer and boil for 2 min to extract the proteins from the beads (*see* **Note 9**).

3.5. Polyacrylamyde Gel Electrophoresis (PAGE)

1. Prepare 16 cm polyacrylamide gels. For instance, 12–14% acrylamide is convenient for analysis of phosphoproteins associated to the TCR-CD3 complex.

2. Load the immunoprecipitates and migrate at 120 V, or at 20 mA/gel constant current.

3.6. Western-Blotting

1. Prepare the PVDF membrane by sinking it first in 15 mL of 100% ethanol, rinse with distilled water, and equilibrate in transfer buffer.

2. Mount the gel and the membrane into the transfer apparatus, according to the manufacturer's instructions.

3. Transfer at 30 V over night, or at 100 V, for 1 h at 4°C. Use a magnetic stirrer to continuously mix transfer buffer (*see* **Note 10**).

4. Check the efficiency of transfer by staining the membrane with

Ponceau S dye for 10 min. Rinse with distilled water until background disappears and protein bands are clearly visible.

5. Remove Ponceau staining by extensive rinsing of the membrane in distilled water.

3.7. Immunodetection of Western Blots

1. Saturate the membrane with Western blotting membrane blocking buffer for 1 h at room temperature on a tilting shaker.
2. Rinse twice for 5 min with Western washing buffer.
3. Incubate with anti-phosphotyrosine MAb, 4G10 at 0.5 µg/mL in Western blotting Ab incubation buffer, for 1 h at room temperature on a tilting shaker.
4. Wash four times for at least 10 min each with Western blotting washing buffer
5. Incubate with horseradish peroxidase-linked goat anti-mouse Ab, at the dilution suggested by the manufacturer, for 1 h at room temperature on a tilting shaker (*see* **Note 11**).
6. Wash four times for at least 10 min each with Western blotting washing buffer.
7. Reveal using enhance chemiluminiscence (ECL) reagents following manufacturer's instructions.

4. Notes

1. There exist commercially available ready made cocktails of protease inhibitors and phosphatase inhibitors (Sigma) that can replace the addition of various single inhibitor solutions.
2. Originally, Western blotting transfer buffer was made with methanol. For safety reasons (methanol is neurotoxic), methanol has been replaced by ethanol with very good transfer results.
3. Fetal calf serum (FCS) is removed in this step of the experiment to avoid cell activation by growth factors from the serum, which may increase the background of phosphoproteins and therefore reduce the differences in protein tyrosine phosphorylation between cells activated with superantigen and controls.
4. The T cell-APC ratio used can be of 1 or be reduced to 2 or even to 3. This allows for some of the experiments to reduce the background of phosphoproteins coming from the APCs. We have observed that Raji

cells display some tyrosine phosphorylated polypeptides that may perturb the analysis of phosphorylation for some particular proteins.

5. The experiment described here with the tumor T-cell line Jurkat, can be also performed with peripheral blood T lymphocytes. In that case, the amounts of cells need to be increased two to five times. Raji can be still be used as APC. Superantigen activation can be performed in this case with a cocktail of *Staphylococcus aureus* enterotoxins composed of SEA, SEB, SEC2, SEE and TSST-1 at 2 µg/mL each.

6. Centrifugation of cell lysates at 13,000 for 15 min removes undesirable background proteins. However, it must be kept in mind that it may also remove part of the proteins of interest, if they are linked to the cytoskeleton. It may also remove detergent-insoluble membrane microdomains, which are rich in T-cell activatory proteins. This type of centrifugation may be replaced by a low-speed 800g for 10 min centrifugation meant to remove mainly nuclei.

7. Irrelevant Abs can be commercially available. Suitable ones would be immunoglobulins of the same isotype than that used for immunoprecipitation. We often used other irrelevant Abs, such as an anti-beta-galatosidase. When immunoprecipitations are carried out with an antiserum, the irrelevant Ab may be a pre-immune serum.

8. Protein-A does not bind with equal affinity to all Ig isotypes. Typically, it binds well to mouse IgG2 but poorly to mouse IgG1. If the Ab used is a mouse monoclonal of the IgG1 isotype, its binding to protein A should be tested or protein-A replaced by protein-G sepharose beads.

9. Under the conditions described here, elution of immunoprecipitation beads will also elute the Ab used for immunopreciptation, giving a strong band in Western blots at 50 kDa. It is the Ig heavy chain that is detected by the secondary Abs. If this band perturbs the detection of a protein of interest, the Abs may be precoupled to protein-A sepharose beads and chemically cross-linked to the beads using dimethylpimelimidate. This avoids the strong elution of Ig.

10. Although transfer in 1 h may be more convenient than overnight transfer, some proteins transfer more efficiently by overnight transfer.

11. Avoid excess of Abs, since this may increase more the background than the specific signal. Primary Ab solutions, such those of the anti-phosphotyrosine MAb 4G10, can be recycled up to five times. In this case, add 0.05% sodium azide to avoid bacterial contamination. However, avoid sodium azide in horseradish peroxidase-coupled secondary Abs, since azide inhibits peroxidase activity.

References

1. Kappler, J., Kotzin, B., Herron, L., Gelfand, E. W., Bigler, R. D., Boylston, A., et al. (1989) V$_\beta$-specific stimulation of human T-cells by staphylococcal toxins. *Science* **24,** 811–814.
2. Niedergang, F., Dautry-Varsat, A., and Alcover, A. (1998) Cooperative activation of TCRs by enterotoxin superantigens. *J. Immunol.* **161,** 6054–6058.
3. Acuto, O. and Cantrell, D. (2000) T cell activation and the cytoskeleton. *Ann. Rev. Immunol.* **18,** 165–184.
4. Zhang, W. and Samelson, L. E. (2000) The role of membrane-associated adaptors in T cell receptor signalling. *Semin. Immunol.* **12,** 35–41.

10

Measurement of Proinflammatory Cytokines and T-Cell Proliferative Response in Superantigen-Activated Human Peripheral Blood Mononuclear Cells

Teresa Krakauer

1. Introduction

The bacterial superantigens, toxic shock syndrome toxin 1 (TSST-1) and the distantly related staphylococcal enterotoxin A and B (SEA and SEB) are potent stimulators of the immune system and cause a variety of diseases in humans, ranging from food poisoning, autoimmune diseases, and toxic shock *(1,2)*.

These superantigens bind directly to major histocompatibility complex (MHC) class II molecules on antigen-presenting cells (APCs) *(2,3)* and specific V_β regions of the T-cell antigen receptors *(4)*. These staphylococcal exotoxins polyclonally activate large populations of T cells. Stimulated monocytes/macrophages and T cells produce massive amounts of proinflammatory cytokines and chemokines *(2,5)*. Previous studies demonstrated that the cytokines produced tumor-necrosis factor-α (TNF-α), interleukin 1 (IL-1), and interferon-γ (IFN-γ) are pathogenic at high concentrations in vivo. TNF-α and IL-1 act synergistically with IFN-γ to enhance immune reactions and promote tissue injury *(6)*. TNF-α, in particu-

From: *Methods in Molecular Biology, vol. 214: Superantigen Protocols*
Edited by: T. Krakauer © Humana Press Inc., Totowa, NJ

lar was identified as the key mediator of toxic shock and anti-TNF-α antibodies had a protective effect in SEB-induced lethal toxic shock *(7,8)*. Thus inhibition of the cytokine cascade may represent a therapeutic approach to mitigate superantigen (SAg)-induced toxic shock.

Described here are simple methods for the quantitation of TNF-α and IFN-γ from the supernatants of TSST-1-stimulated human peripheral blood mononuclear cells (PBMC) by enzyme-linked immunosorbent assay (ELISA). A bioassay of T-cell proliferation in response to TSST-1 is also presented to assess the polyclonal activation of T cells by superantigen. The response of PBMC to LPS, which is not a superantigen and activates cells through toll-like receptors, is included as a comparison to the superantigen TSST-1. Attenuation of T cell proliferation and proinflammatory cytokine production by TSST-1-stimulated human PBMC by tricyclodecan-9-yl (D609), an inhibitor of phosphatidylcholine-specific phospholipase C, was used to illustrate the utility of these assays in the screening of anti-inflammatory drugs.

2. Materials

2.1. Peripheral Blood Mononuclear Cell Culture

1. Human peripheral blood collected in heparinized tubes. Keep at room temperature (20°C) until used. Sodium heparin 1000 U/mL.
2. Ficoll-Paque (Pharmacia, Piscataway, NJ).
3. Culture medium: RPMI 1640, 10% heat-inactivated fetal calf serum (FCS), 100 U/mL penicillin, 100 µg/mL streptomycin, and 2 mM L-glutamine (all from Life Technologies, Gaithersburg, MD).
4. Purified TSST-1 (Toxin Technology, Sarasota, FL).
5. Lipopolysaccharide (LPS) *E. coli* 055:B5 (Difco, Detroit, MI), optional reagent.
6. Tricyclodecan-9-yl xanthogenate (D609) (Alexis, Milwaukee, WI), optional reagent.
7. 24-well cell culture plates (Corning-Costar).

2.2. Detection and Quantitation of TNF-α by ELISA

1. Recombinant human (h) TNF-α (Boehringer-Mannheim, Indianapolis, IN).
2. Monoclonal antibody (Mab) to hTNF-α (Boehringer-Mannheim).
3. Polyclonal goat anti-h TNF-α (R and D Systems, Minneapolis, MN).
4. Peroxidase-conjugated swine anti-goat IgG (Boehringer-Mannheim)
5. Chromogen TMB substrate solution: equal volumes of 3,3',5,5'-tetramethylbenzidine (TMB) solution and H_2O_2 (Kirkegaard and Perry, Gaithersburg, MD) prepared immediately fresh before use.
6. Stop solution: $2 N H_2SO_4$.
7. Wash buffer: Phosphate-buffered saline (PBS), pH 7.4 (Sigma, St. Louis, MO), 0.05% Tween-20.
8. Blocking solution 1: 1% bovine serum albumin (BSA) in PBS.
9. 96-well Maxisorp Nunc plates.
10. ELISA plate reader (Dynatech, Chantilly, VA).

2.3. Detection and Quantitation of IFN-γ by ELISA

1. Recombinant h IFN-γ (Collaborative Research, Bedford, MA).
2. Monoclonal antibody to h IFN-γ (Interferon Science, New Brunswick, NJ).
3. Biotinylated anti-h IFN-γ (Pharmingen, San Diego, CA).
4. Peroxidase-streptavidin (Kirkegaard and Perry)
5. Chromogen TMB solution, same as above for TNF-α ELISA.
6. Stop solution: $2 N H_2SO_4$.
7. Wash buffer, same as above for TNF-α ELISA.
8. Blocking solution 2: 2% BSA, 0.05% Tween-20 in PBS.

2.4. Measurement of T-Cell Proliferation

1. ^{3}H-Thymidine, specific activity of 2 Ci/mmol (Amersham, Arlington Heights, IL).
2. PBMC culture medium, same as for PBMC culture.
3. 96-well flat bottom plate with low evaporation lid (Corning-Costar).
4. 96-well plate harvester (Packard or Skatron).

5. β-scintillation counter, for example, 1205 Betaplate Counter (Pharmacia LKB Nuclear, Gaithersburg, MD).

3. Methods

3.1. Culture of Human PBMC

3.1.1. Separation of Human PBMC

PBMC are obtained from peripheral blood by differential gradient centrifugation over Ficoll-Paque. Sterile cell cultureware and reagents are used for cell culture and T-cell proliferation. Aseptic procedures are used in a laminar flow hood.

1. Place 20 mL of Ficoll-Paque at the bottom of a 50 mL polycarbonate centrifuge tube.
2. Pipet 25–30 mL of heparinized blood carefully onto Ficoll–Paque layer (*see* **Note 1**).
3. Centrifuge at 300*g* for 20 min.
4. PBMC band at the interphase and appear as a cloudy layer above Ficoll-Paque layer. Collect PBMC with pipet carefully and transfer cells to a 50-mL tube (*see* **Note 2**).
5. Wash cells twice with RPMI 1640 or PBS and pellet cells at 250*g* for 10 min.
6. Resuspend PBMC in 10 mL of culture medium. Count cells and readjust cells to 2×10^6 cells/mL.

3.1.2. PBMC Culture

1. A well with PBMC and culture medium alone serves as a background negative control. The final volume of each culture is 1 mL at 1×10^6 cells/mL. Additional wells can be prepared with different superantigens and stimulants of interest. TSST-1 is used as an example here.
2. Add 100 μL of TSST-1 (1.5 μg/mL) to a 24-well cell culture plate. A dose-response curve can be obtained by preparing different dilutions of TSST-1 from a stock solution of 1 mg/mL. Usually 10–200 ng/mL of TSST-1 represents an optimal range.
3. Additional wells of other agents, either stimulants (LPS) or inhibi-

tors, can be prepared. For example, 100 μL of D609 (2 mM), the inhibitor to be tested is added in the presence or absence of TSST-1.

4. 0.5 mL of PBMC (2×10^6 cells/mL) is added to each well.

5. Additional volume of culture medium is added to a final volume of 1 mL (*see* **Note 3**).

6. Cells are incubated at 37°C in a 5% CO_2 incubator.

7. Supernatants are harvested from these cultures after 16 h and store frozen until use (*see* **Note 4**).

3.2. Detection of TNF-α by ELISA

TNF-α can be detected in culture supernatants by ELISA. The choice of ELISA format and reagents is at the discretion of the investigator. ELISA kits, MAbs and PAbs to TNF-α and other cytokines and chemokines are commercially available (*see* **Note 5**). In general commercial ELISA kits are not reliable between different lots and therefore not recommended for comparing serial samples in a longitudinal study collected over months or years (*see* **Note 6**). Furthermore, different and multiple diluents are used for standard, assay samples, and antibodies and one cannot be sure what is in these solutions that make an assay work and whether samples and standards are "treated" equally in these ELISA kits. Also, if an investigator is interested in studying multiple cytokines and chemokines, it is easier to keep one wash buffer, one blocking solution and one diluent instead of five different sets of wash buffers, blocking solutions, and diluents for five different cytokines for these ELISA kits. The ELISA Guidebook in the Molecular Biology Protocols series describes the theory and practice of ELISA (*9*), as well as preparation of antibodies and conjugates in detail. The method described here for TNF-α is an indirect sandwich ELISA using capture antibody, tested sample (supernatant), second anti-cytokine antibody, peroxidase conjugated anti-second anti-cytokine antibody, and chromogen.

1. Add 100 μL of 5 μg/mL monoclonal anti-TNF-α to each well of ELISA plate. Incubate at 37°C for 2 h to coat plate (*see* **Note 7**).

2. Aspirate each well and wash with wash buffer three times (*see* **Notes**

8 and **9**). At this point, plates can be stored in Zip-Lock bags for 2 wk at 4°C or be used immediately (*see* **Note 10**).

3. On the day of ELISA, block plates by adding 200 µL of blocking buffer 1. Incubate plate for 1 h at 37°C. Aspirate and discard block buffer. Blot plate on absorbent paper towel to remove residual blocking buffer.

4. Prepare a set of TNF-α standards for calibration (*see* **Note 11**). The solution used for dilution of the standard should be consistent with the samples (supernatants) to be tested for the presence of TNF-α. Serial dilutions of TNF-α are prepared in culture medium. Add 100 µL of culture medium as background control to the first two wells. Add 100 µL of each TNF-α standards (20–1000 ng/mL) and culture supernatants from PBMC culture in duplicate. Incubate plate 2 h at 37°C.

5. Wash plate three times with wash buffer, blot off excess wash on absorbent paper towel (*see* **Note 12**).

6. Add 100 µL of goat anti-human TNF-α (0.83 µg/mL in blocking buffer 1) to each well (*see* **Note 13**). Incubate 1.75 h at 37°C.

7. Wash plate three times with wash buffer (*see* **Note 12**).

8. Add 100 µL of peroxidase-congugated swine anti-goat IgG (1/2000 dilution in blocking buffer 1) (*see* **Note 14**). Incubate 20 min at 37°C.

9. Wash plate four times with wash buffer (*see* **Note 12**).

10. Add 100 µL of chromogen TBM solution to each well. At this point, color development (blue-green) is observed visually for > 5 min depending on how fast color develops. The ELISA plate is placed on plate reader and OD readings are obtained at 630 nm (*see* **Note 15**).

11. Add 100 µL of 2 *N* stop solution to each well to stop further color development. Color will turn yellow at this point. Place plate on plate reader and record OD at 450 nm at 5 min after adding stop solution (*see* **Note 15**).

12. Generate a standard curve from OD readings of TNF-α standards using linear regression. Use this to calculate levels of TNF-α in unknown samples (*see* **Note 16**).

Figure 1 shows the levels of TNF-α from TSST-1- and LPS-stimulated cultures. Both TSST-1 and LPS induced high and comparable levels of TNF-α from PBMC. The phospholipase C inhibitor, D609 at 0.2 m*M*, completely inhibited TNF-α release from stimulated PBMC (*see* **Fig. 1**)

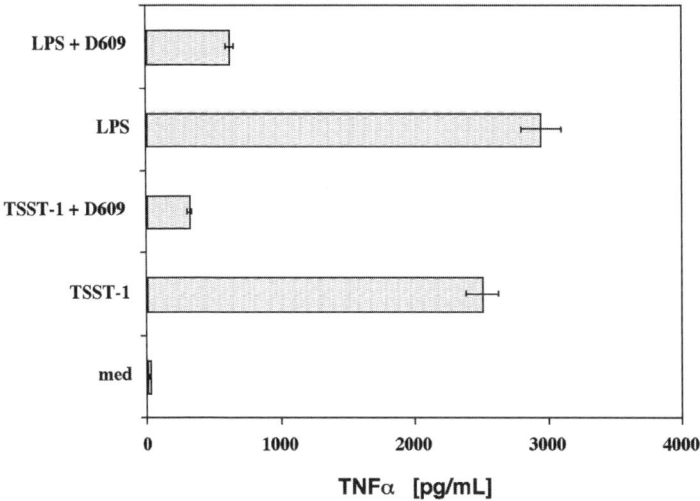

Fig. 1. Inhibition of TNF-α production by PBMC stimulated with TSST-1 (150 ng/mL) or LPS (100 ng/mL) in the presence of 0.2 mM of D609. Values represent the means ± SD of duplicate samples from three experiments.

3.3. Detection of IFN-γ by ELISA

IFN-γ, a product of activated T lymphocytes, can also be detected in the same supernatants of superantigen-stimulated T cells. The ELISA method described here is slightly different from the one used earlier for TNF-α and illustrates a general format applicable with biotinylated anti-cytokine antibody. This direct sandwich ELISA method for IFN-γ detection uses capture antibody, sample (supernatants), biotinylated second anti-cytokine antibody, peroxidase-streptoavidin, and chromogen substrate.

1. Add 100 µL of 25 neutralizing U/mL monoclonal anti-IFN-γ to each well of ELISA plate. Incubate at 37°C for 2 h to coat plate (*see* **Note 7**).
2. Aspirate each well and wash with wash buffer three times (*see* **Notes 8** and **9**). At this point, plates can be stored in zip-lock bags or used immediately (*see* **Note 10**).
3. On the day of ELISA, block plates by adding 200 µL of blocking buffer 2. Incubate 1 h at 37°C. Aspirate and discard block buffer (*see* **Note 12**).

4. Prepare a set of IFN-γ standards (20–1000 ng/mL) for calibration in the same way as TNF-α (**step 5** of **Subheading 3.2.**). Add 100 μL of culture medium as background control or each IFN-γ standards in duplicate. Add threefold or more diluted supernatants from PBMC culture (*see* **Note 17**). Incubate plate 2 h at 37°C.

5. Wash plate three times with wash buffer (*see* **Note 12**).

6. Add 100 μL of biotinylated anti-human IFN-γ (0.5 μg/mL in blocking buffer 2) to each well. Incubate 45 min at 37°C.

7. Wash plate four times with wash buffer (*see* **Note 12**).

8. Add 100 μL of peroxidase-streptoavidin (1/600) dilution in blocking buffer 2). Incubate 30 min at 37°C.

9. Wash plate four times with wash buffer (*see* **Note 12**).

10. Add 100 μL of chromogen TBM solution to each well. Follow color development (blue-green) visually for 5 min. Place ELISA plate on plate reader and obtain OD readings at 630 nm (*see* **Note 15**).

11. Add 100 μL of 2 *N* stop solution to each well to stop further color development. Read plate at 450 nm at 5 min after adding stop solution (*see* **Note 15**).

12. Generate a standard curve from OD readings of IFN-γ standards using linear regression. Use this curve to determine levels of IFN-γ in unknown samples (*see* **Note 16**).

Figure 2 shows that the superantigen, TSST-1, induced high levels of IFN-γ, whereas LPS which was not a superantigen, is a poor activator for IFN-γ. D609 suppressed TSST-1-induced IFN-γ by 75%.

3.4. T-Cell Proliferation Assay

T-cell activation is a hallmark of superantigen activation. A simple inexpensive method to detect this activation is by the incorporation of ^{3}H-thymidine into proliferating T cells. The setup of this assay is similar to that of PBMC culture, except microwells (in 96-well plate) are used and each parameter is in triplicate.

1. Three wells with PBMC and culture medium alone serve as background negative control. The final volume of each culture is 0.2 mL at 1×10^6 cells/mL (*see* **Note 18**).

2. Add 50 μL of TSST-1 (600 ng/mL) to each well of a 96-well tissue-culture plate. A dose-response curve can be obtained by preparing

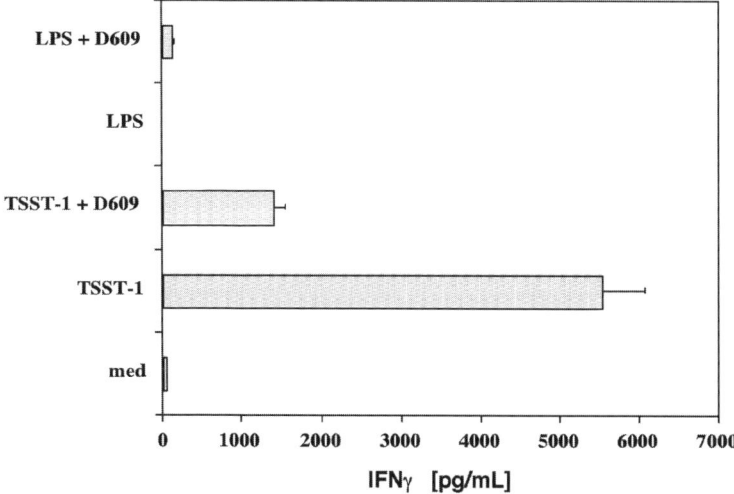

Fig. 2. Inhibition of IFN-γ production by PBMC stimulated with TSST-1 (150 ng/mL) or LPS (100 ng/mL) in the presence of 0.2 mM of D609. Values represent the means ± SD of duplicate samples from three experiments.

different dilutions of TSST-1 from a stock solution of 1 mg/mL. Usually 10–200 ng/mL of TSST-1 represents an optimal range.

3. Additional wells of other agents, either stimulants or inhibitors, can be prepared. For example, 50 μL of D609 (0.8 mM), the inhibitor to be tested, is added in the presence or absence of TSST-1.

4. 100 μL of PBMC (2×10^6 cells/mL) is added to each well.

5. Additional volume (50 μL) of culture medium is added to a final volume of 0.2 mL/well. Tap plate gently to mix reagents.

6. Cells are incubated at 37°C in a 5% CO_2 incubator.

7. After 2 d (usually at 40 h, in the morning of d 2), 10 μL of 2 mCi/mL ^{3}H-thymidine in culture medium is added to each well. Tap plate gently to mix reagents. Incubate plate at 37°C in a 5% CO_2 incubator for an additional 5–6 h (*see* **Note 19**).

8. Harvest plate with a harvester and collect incorporated ^{3}H-thymidine onto filter paper. Count ^{3}H-thymidine with a β-scintillation counter.

A typical T-cell proliferation assay for TSST-1 and LPS is shown in **Fig. 3**.

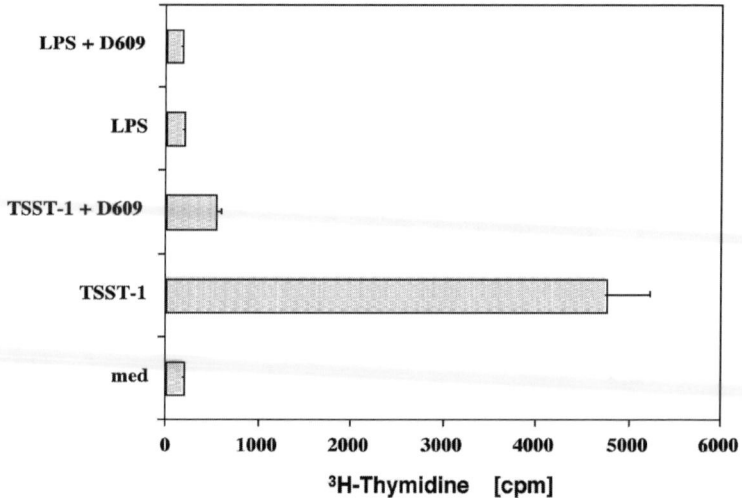

Fig. 3. Inhibition of TSST-1-induced T-cell proliferation By D609.
PBMC were stimulated with TSST-1 (150 ng/mL) or LPS (100 ng/mL) in
the presence or absence of 0.2 m*M* D609. Values are the means ± SD of
triplicate cultures and represent three experiments.

4. Notes

1. Avoid mixing blood into Ficoll-Paque layer at the bottom of the tube
   to get a good "band" of PBMC after centrifugation. This can be
   accomplished by pointing pipet tip onto the side of tube when deliv-
   ering blood onto the gradient.
2. Minimize erythrocyte (at the bottom of centrifuge tube) contamination at this stage of collecting PBMC.
3. One can scale up to 1.2 mL of total volume without changing the
   conditions extensively. Avoid filling to 2 mL/well as crowding of
   cells occurs and it is hard to mix reagents in a full well without spill-
   ing its contents.
4. Supernatants can be harvested at 48 h or longer. However, most of
   the critical cytokines except for TNF-β, peak at 16–24 h.
5. There are many advantages in devising your own ELISA for
   cytokines. Assays are more reproducible and cost less. One can cus-
   tomize and create a similar format of ELISA for different cytokines
   so that multiple ELISA for different cytokines can be performed
   together, saving time.

6. ELISA plates are fresh and ready to go when assays are needed because one can plan the coating of ELISA plates better. Commercial ELISA kits usually have a short shelf-life.

7. Preventing evaporation of plates is critical for reproducibility of results and assuring uniformity of wells on the edges of the plate with the rest. This can be achieved by placing another ELISA plate on top of assay plate. This plate can be reused repeatedly as a cover.

8. A simple, hand-held, 12-well manifold dispenser can be used.

9. Avoid using sodium azide in wash buffers or diluents as it inhibits peroxidase activity.

10. Plates can be stored in Zip-Lock bags for 2 wk or more. However, best results are obtained with fresh plates.

11. Cytokine standard stock solution for calibrating ELISA should be at >1 µg/mL and kept at –20°C or –70°C for long- term storage. Distribute cytokine stock solution into small aliquots (5–20 µL) to avoid multiple freeze-thaw cycles.

12. For each wash, it is important to fill each well with >200 µL of wash buffer, remove wash buffer, and invert plate to drain off wash buffer completely on absorbent paper towel between washes. High background and poor reproducibility of replicates generally result from inadequate washing. Increasing the number of washes to five might help in some cases. Blot off excess liquid between washes on paper towels.

13. Antibody stock solution should be stored undiluted until use, at the manufacturer's suggested concentration and temperature.

14. Try a different concentration of detecting antibody if no signal or high background is observed. Titrate antibody pairs again if this fails. We have used one lot of anti-goat antibody requiring a 1/20,000 dilution instead of the ususal 1/2000. Increasing the number of washes and lowering the concentrations of detecting antibodies would help to lower high background OD.

15. After adding TMB chromogen substrate to ELISA plate, monitor color development carefully. The OD reading should not be allowed to exceed 0.4 OD units because the addition of stop solution results in fourfold increases in OD values when read at 450 nm. Most plate readers (spectrophotometer) are not sensitive at >1.6 OD. Use a lower concentration of conjugate antibody if color develops too fast.

16. The range of standards can be minimized or extended depending on the levels of cytokines present in stimulated cell supernatants. PBMC from some donors are activated to produce higher levels than others.

Five to six dilutions of standards from 20–1000 pg/mL should be used. Pairs of cytokine antibodies (coating antibody and detecting antibody) should be titrated against each other to optimize the assay. A checkerboard format should be used when titrating these antibodies to obtain the best signal to noise ratio for a given standard range. Antibodies vary from lot to lot and restandardization is necessary when a new lot or bottle is used. It is generally difficult to cover >3 log concentration of standard and still maintain a strong signal, minimum background, and a linear standard curve.

17. Diluted supernatants (in culture medium) can be used when IFN-γ is present in large amounts.

18. Higher number of cells can be used to increase signal.

19. The incubation period for ^{3}H-thymidine can be increased to 16 h to accommodate the schedule of the investigator. Background might increase a little with longer incubation time.

20. A general comment on ELISA antibodies to avoid pitfalls. Different batches of antibodies and conjugates from the same manufacturer may vary. Thus, in large-scale applications, it is good practice to obtain a sufficient batch of an antibody for all future testing. Anti-cytokine antibodies vary tremendously from different companies in terms of epitope specificity, affinities, and therefore reactivity. It is useful to screen a couple of antibodies from different sources for a backup. Conjugates must be titrated to optimum conditions and not be used in excess.

References

1. Kotzin, B. L., Leung, D. Y. M., Kappler, J., and Marrack, P. A. (1993) Superantigens and their potential role in human disease. *Adv. Immunol.* **54,** 99–166.

2. Schlievert, P. M. (1993) Role of superantigens in human disease. *J. Infect. Dis.* **167,** 997–1002.

3. Choi, Y., Kotzin, B., Hernon, L., Callahan, J., Marrack, P., and Kappler, J. (1989) Interaction of *Staphylococcus aureus* toxin "superantigens" with human T cells. *Proc. Natl. Acad. Sci. USA* **86,** 8941–8945.

4. Gascoigne, N. R. J. and Ames K. T. (1991) Direct binding of secreted TCR β chain to superantigen associated with MHC class II complex protein. *Proc. Natl. Acad. Sci. USA* **88,** 613–616.

5. Jupin, C., Anderson, S., Damais, C., Alouf, J. E., and Parant, M. (1988) Toxic shock syndrome toxin 1 as an inducer of human tumor necrosis factors and gamma interferon. *J. Exp. Med.* **167,** 752–761.
6. Krakauer, T., Vilcek, J., and Oppenheim, J. J. (1998) Proinflammatory cytokines, in *Fundamental Immunology* (Paul, W., ed.), Lippincott-Raven, Philadephia, PA, pp. 775–811.
7. Miethke, T., Wahl, C., Heeg, K., Echtenacher, B., Krammer, P. B., and Wagner, H. (1992) T cell-mediated lethal shock triggered in mice by the superantigen SEB: critical role of TNF. *J. Exp. Med.* **175,** 91–98.
8. Miethke, T., Wahl, C., Regele, D., Gaus, H., Heeg, K., and Wagner, H. (1993) Superantigen mediated shock: A cytokine release syndrome. *Immunbiology* **189,** 270–284.
9. Crowther, J. R. (ed.) (2000) *ELISA Guidebook.* Humana Press, Totowa, NJ.

11

RNase Protection Assay for the Study of the Differential Effects of Therapeutic Agents in Suppressing Staphylococcal Enterotoxin B-Induced Cytokines in Human Peripheral Blood Mononuclear Cells

Teresa Krakauer, Xin Chen, O. M. Zack Howard, and Howard A. Young

1. Introduction

Staphylococcal exotoxins (SE) are among the most common etiological agents that cause toxic shock *(1)*. Similar to other superantigens, SE activates T cells polyclonally by binding simultaneously to specific V_β regions of T-cell receptors (TCR) on T cells and the major histocompatibility complex class II (MHC II) molecules on antigen-presenting cells (APCs) *(2,3)*. Interaction of SE with TCR and MHC II results in a massive release of proinflammatory cytokines from stimulated cells *(4,5)*. Previous studies demonstrated that the cytokines produced, tumor-necrosis factor (TNF-α), interleukin 1 (IL-1), and interferon-γ (IFN-γ) are pivotal mediators in SE-induced toxic shock *(6,7)*. High levels of these cytokines in serum are pathogenic and correlate with clinical symptoms of toxic shock *(8–10)*.

From: *Methods in Molecular Biology, vol. 214: Superantigen Protocols*
Edited by: T. Krakauer © Humana Press Inc., Totowa, NJ

Because of the central role these cytokines play in the pathogenesis of toxic shock, the regulation of the expression of cytokine mRNA in SE-stimulated human peripheral blood mononuclear cells (PBMC) in the presence of various therapeutic compounds was investigated. We describe here the use of the RNase protection assay (RPA) as a method to probe the in vitro effects of various anti-infectious and anti-inflammatory agents in suppressing staphylococcal enterotoxin B (SEB)-induced cytokine production at the molecular level.

2. Materials

2.1. RNA Preparation from Human PBMC

1. Ficoll-Paque (Pharmacia, Piscataway, NJ).
2. Cell-culture medium: RPMI 1640, 10% heat-inactivated fetal calf serum (FCS), 100 U/mL penicillin, 100 μg/mL streptomycin and 2 mM L-glutamine (all from Life Technologies, Gaithersburg, MD).
3. SEB (Toxin Technology, Sarasota, FL).
4. Tricyclodecan-9-yl xanthogenate D609 (Alexis, Milwaukee, WI), optional test compound.
5. Baicalin (B.Q. Li, USPTO, VA), optional test compound.
6. Chlorogenic acid (Sigma, St. Louis, MO), optional test compound.
7. TRIzol (Invitrogen, Carlsbad, CA).

2.2. RNase Protection Assay

2.2.1. Probe Synthesis Reagents

1. RiboQuant In Vitro Transcription Kit (Cat. no. 556850, Pharmingen, San Diego, CA).
2. ^{33}P-UTP, 3000Ci/mmol (Cat. no. NEG307H, New England Nuclear).
3. Individual components: Pharmingen RiboQuant Multiprobe template sets (Cat. nos. vary).
4. Dithiothreitol (DTT), 100 mM (Cat. no. 45006Z, Pharmingen).
5. Nucleotide mix (Cat. no. 45005Z, Pharmingen).
6. Transcription buffer (Cat. no. 45007A, Pharmingen).
7. T7 RNA polymerase (Cat. no. 45009Z, Pharmingen).

8. Ambion T7 RNA polymerase/RNase Inhibitor Maxiscript (Cat. no. 2086G, Pharmingen).
9. RNase-free DNase I (Cat. no. 45010Z, Pharmingen).
10. MicroSpin G25 columns (Cat. no. 27-5325-01, Amersham, Arlington Heights, IL).

2.2.2. RPA Reagents

1. RNase Protection Assay Kit (Cat. no. 45014K, Pharmingen).
2. RNase A + T1 Mix (Cat. no. 45017Z, Pharmingen).
3. Hybridization buffer (Cat. no. 45015A, Pharmingen).
4. Yeast tRNA (Cat. no. 45011Z, Pharmingen).
5. RPA II RNase inactivation reagent (Cat. no. 8539G, Ambion, Austin, TX).
6. GlycoBlue Coprecipitant (Cat. no. 9515-9516, Ambion).
7. Boekel model 111007 temperature block.

2.2.3. Gel Electrophoresis Reagents

1. Loading buffer (Cat. no. 45022A, Pharmingen).
2. Gel mix 6 (Cat. no. 15543-010. Invitrogen-Life Technologies).
3. Sigmacote (Cat. no. SL-2, Sigma).
4. Kodak BioMax MS X-ray film (Cat. no. 143-5726, VWR Scientific).
5. TransScreen LE Intensifying screen with 1 cassette (Cat. no. 852-7558, VWR Scientific).

3. Methods

3.1. RNA Preparation from Human PBMC

1. Human PBMC are isolated by Ficoll-Paque density gradient centrifugation of heparinized blood from normal human donors as described in Chapter 10.
2. PBMC (2×10^6 cells/mL) are cultured at 37°C in T75 cell culture flask containing (16–30 mL) of RPMI 1640 culture medium and 10% heat-inactivated fetal bovine serum (FBS). Cell culture flasks are placed horizontally for the entire incubation period to allow for the adherence of monocytes and loosely adherent cells. The superantigen, SEB, and various compounds to be tested are added at

10× concentration immediately in sequence after PBMC addition to cell-culture flasks.

3. After incubation for 4 h, the cell-culture flask is set upright and supernatants are removed immediately. Total RNA is isolated from cells remaining in T75 by using 1 mL of cold TRIzol reagent. Flasks are placed horizontally for 5–7 min at room temperature so that TRIzol covers the entire surface area of flask with cells.

4. TRIzol is removed and stored in 2 mL polycarbonate vials at –70°C until use.

3.2. RNase Protection Assay

The ribonuclease protection assay (RPA) is a sensitive and quantitative method to assay levels of gene transcripts. Although not as sensitive as reverse transcription polymerase chain reaction (RT-PCR), this method is more easily quantitated and far more sensitive than Northern blots. Furthermore with the commercialization of Multiprobe template kits, this assay can now be utilized to measure the relative levels of 8–10 genes by using as little as 1 µg of total cellular RNA.

The RPA utilizes the bacteriophage polymerases T7 or SP6. The recognition sequences for these polymerases are highly specific and, when inserted in front of target genes, permit in vitro transcription of RNAs representing either the sense or anti-sense strand of the RNA *(11,12)*. For use in the RPA, an antisense transcript is synthesized containing a radiolabeled UTP molecule incorporated into the transcript and then hybridized to total cellular RNA or poly A+ RNA. Note that the in vitro synthesized transcript also contains a small number (e.g., 50–70) nucleotides from the plasmid template. These extra nucleotides will not be protected by the cellular RNA and will serve to distinguish the template RNA from the protected RNA. If the target mRNA is present in the cell, a double-stranded RNA molecule is formed during the hybridization step. The hybridization reaction is then digested with a combination of RNases A and T1. These RNases digest any single-strand RNA while the duplex RNA is protected from digestion. After inactivation of the RNase cocktail, the protected RNA is precipitated, resuspended, heated to 90°C and run on a denaturing polyacrylamide gel. In the Multiprobe Template kits available commercially from Pharmingen, 8–10 templates are included in a single template set and are all labeled in a single reaction. Note that the templates are all designed to cross exons, thus reducing any problem with contaminating DNA. The first Multiprobe template systems analyzed T-cell receptor (TCR) gene expression *(13,14)* and an example of how to generate templates not commercially available was recently published *(15)*. Also, two laboratories have reported that the use of the commercially template sets can lead to misinterpretation of data owing to unexpected polymorphisms found in specific strains of mice *(16,17)*.

3.2.1. Probe Synthesis

Probe synthesis is generally carried out today with the use of commercially available In Vitro Transcription Kits. The major suppliers are Pharmingen, Ambion, and Promega.

1. The kits contain the reaction buffer, nucleotide mix (minus UTP), RNAsin (an RNase inhibitor), DTT, the T7 polymerase (*see* **Note 1**), RNase-free DNAse Ia carrier yeast tRNA and EDTA as a stop buffer (*see* **Note 2**). The advantage of using a kit is that all reagents are tested to work well together.
2. 70–100 µCi of either ^{32}P-UTP or ^{33}P-UTP is included in the reaction.
3. The reaction (20 µL) is incubated at 37°C for 60 min (*see* **Notes 3** and **4**), followed by the addition of DNAse I for 30 min at 37°C to digest the template DNAs (*see* **Notes 5–8**).
4. 4 µg of yeast tRNA carrier is added as well as an equal volume (23 µL) of 20 m*M* EDTA (*see* **Notes 9** and **10**).

3.2.2. Probe Purification

One manufacturer recommends phenol-chloroform extraction and isopropanol precipitation as a method of preparing the probe for hybridization. However, this generates radioactive organic waste and thus should be avoided.

1. Probes are more easily purified away from free isotope by using the Amersham MicroSpin G25 columns (Cat. no. 27-5325-01).

2. After a 1-min centrifugation to remove the column buffer (*see* **Note 11**), the entire reaction is placed onto the column followed by a short 2 min centrifugation to elute the labeled probes.

3. Count 1 µL of the probe. Use scintillation fluid if counting ^{33}P but with ^{32}P, save scintillation fluid and count 1 µL without fluid (Cerenkov counting). Just be sure to know the ratio of cpms with and without scintillation fluid for your particular scintillation counter.

3.2.3. Hybridization

Hybridization consists of adding the target RNA, radiolabeled anti-sense RNA probes and a hybridization buffer containing formamide. Once again both Pharmingen and Ambion make kits with all necessary reagents for hybridization and processing of the RNA-RNA hybrids.

1. RNA is added to 10–12 µL of hybridization buffer for most reactions (*see* **Note 12**). It is relatively important to maintain at least 50–75% hybridization buffer. The reaction volume is kept below 20 µL but up to 40 µL can be used when the RNA is very dilute. Generally, the RNA concentration is 2–5 µg/µL (*see* **Notes 13** and **14**). It is very convenient to make a cocktail of the probe mixed with the hybridization buffer. This permits adding the same amount of probe and hybridization buffer to each RNA (*see* **Note 15**). Mix the RNA, probe and hybridization buffer well by pipetting up and down four to five times.

2. Next, add one drop of mineral oil and place in a 90°C temperature block (Boekel model 111007) (*see* **Note 16**). When the temperature returns to 90°C, turn down to 56°C. Incubate at 56°C overnight. The temperature block you use should get down to 56°C within about 1 h (*see* **Notes 17** and **18**).

3.2.4. RNase Treatment

1. The second day, place hybridization reactions at 37°C for 10–15 min.
2. Add 100 µL of RNase buffer ONLY to control #2.
3. Make cocktail of RNase buffer + RNase (6 µL RNase A + T1 mixture/2.5 mL RNase buffer if using the Pharmingen hybridization kit). Use 100 µL/tube. Mix well by flicking with finger. Place in minifuge for 1–2 min. Incubate at 30°C for 45 min (*see* **Notes 19** and **20**).

3.3.5. Inactivation/Precipitation

Complete inactivation of the RNases is critical. As the RNA hybrid is denatured before gel electrophoresis, all RNases must be inactivated to prevent degradation during the electrophoresis step.

1. To inactivate the RNases, make a master cocktail containing 200 µL of Ambion RNase inactivation reagent (RPA II #8539G), 50 µL of ethanol, 5 µg of yeast tRNA and 1 µL of Ambion GycoBlue co-precipitate (mix this well before pipetting) per RNA sample (*see* **Notes 21–23**). Add 250 µL to 1.5-mL microcentrifuge tubes. Do this during the time the samples are being treated with RNase. The samples are under mineral oil during the hybridization and RNase step so carefully remove the samples, pipet them into the inactivation cocktail and then spot the excess mineral oil onto blotting paper so it becomes solid radioactive waste. Mix the samples and inactivation cocktail by inverting three to four times.
2. Keep the samples at –70°C for 15 min (*see* **Notes 24** and **25**).
3. Centrifuge 15 min in a room temperature microcentrifuge at 20,000g. Carefully pour off the radioactive supernatant, and use a sterile cotton swap to remove excess liquid from the tube (being careful to avoid the blue pellet) (*see* **Notes 26** and **27**).
4. Resuspend the pellet in 3 µL of the Pharmingen sample buffer by pipetting up and down 5–10×. There is no need to wash the pellet (*see* **Notes 28–23**).

3.3.6. Gel Electrophoresis

We use a standard DNA sequencing gel to separate the protected probes (*see* **Notes 34–38**). When using the Multiprobe template sets, the protected probes can range in size from 100 nucleotides to 400 nucleotides. In general, we find that 30 lanes per gel is adequate for most experiments. Don't forget to heat the samples to 90°C before loading the gel. After electrophoresis, gels are dried and exposed to film at –70°C.

A representative RNase protection assay is presented in **Fig. 1**. D609, a phospholipase C inhibitor and the plant flavonoid baicalin inhibit SEB-induced TNF-α mRNA transcript, whereas the plant polyphenol chlorogenic acid has no effect on TNF-α mRNA levels.

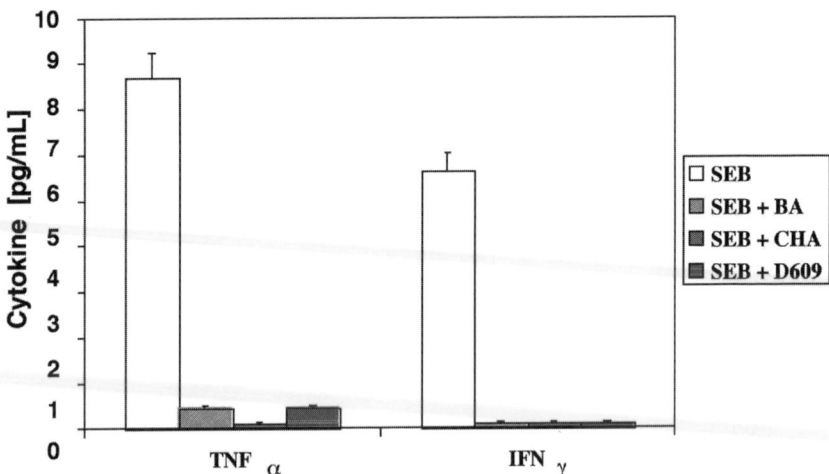

Fig. 1. Inhibition of TNF-α and IFN-γ production by PBMC stimulated with SEB (150 ng/mL) alone or in the presence of 0.2 m*M* D609, or 100 µg/mL baicalin (BA), or 200 µg/mL chloorogenic acid (CHA). Values represent the mean ± standard errors of the means of duplicate samples and represent three experiments. Results are statistically significant (*p* < 0.02) between SEB and SEB plus drug-treated samples.

D609 is the best inhibitor of both TNF-α and IFN-γ mRNA from SEB-stimulated cells. In contrast, all three compounds inhibit TNF-α levels in SEB-stimulated PBMC (*see* **Fig. 2**). These results from RPA demonstrate different modes of inhibition of TNF-α by these inhibitors.

4. Notes

1. We have substituted Ambion T7 polymerase in the Pharmingen synthesis kit with good results.
2. You can add your own probe to a Pharmingen Multiprobe template set. Be sure the protected band falls at a different place than the other bands and add 5–10 ng/probe of synthesis reaction (you may have to titer in your added template) and that the probe crosses two exons of the gene. Clone your gene of interest in a vector that has a T7 polymerase promoter and check the clones to choose one that is the proper orientation to give you an anti-sense transcript. Linearize your plas-

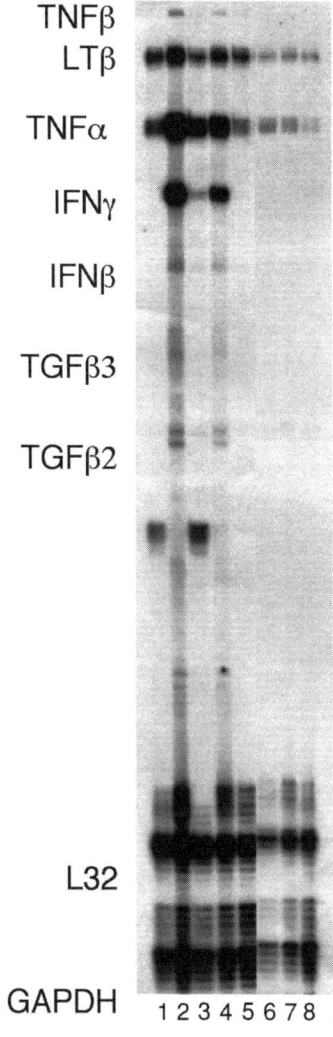

TNFβ
LTβ
TNFα
IFNγ
IFNβ
TGFβ3
TGFβ2
L32
GAPDH 1 2 3 4 5 6 7 8

Fig. 2. Multiprobe RNase protection analysis of TNF-α and IFN-γ mRNA. Total RNA was extracted from human PBMC treated for 4 h with SEB in the presence or absence 100 μg/mL baicalin, or 200 μg/mL chlorogenic acid, or 0.2 m*M* D609. Five μg of total RNA was applied per lane. Lanes 1–8 represent cells in medium alone, SEB-stimulated cells, SEB-stimulated cells plus BA, SEB-stimulated cells plus CHA, SEB-stimulated cells plus D609, cells with BA, cells with CHA, and cells with D609, respectively. Data represent experiments repeated at least three times.

mid at the end of the target gene so that the transcription does not continue through the plasmid DNA. Gel purify your linearized plasmid before use.

3. We have incubated the reaction for 90 min at 37°C as we get an improved labeling with some Multiprobe template sets.

4. Reaction volume can be cut in half successfully to save on isotope. This is worthwhile if you have only 10–15 RNAs to analyze.

5. Do *not* use UTP that contains the colored stabilization reagent, despite what the isotope manufacturers may claim. The reagent inhibits the T7 polymerase.

6. We have successfully used ^{33}P-UTP that is 3 wk past its expiration date although the fresh isotope gives better total yield of labeled probe.

7. If you use ^{32}P-UTP, you must use the probe in 24–36 h. ^{33}P probes are good for at least 4 d.

8. Regarding the use of ^{33}P, be sure you have the proper Geiger counter to detect the isotope. We use one with a "pancake" head. Not all Geiger counters used for ^{32}P are suitable for ^{33}P.

9. You can purchase your yeast tRNA from other sources. However, you may want to extract it with phenol-chloroform, precipitate the RNA, and resuspend in RNase-free H_2O before use.

10. Buy backup vials of just about everything. It can be a disaster if you are in the middle of everything and you run out of a reagent.

11. When spinning the G25 columns to remove the buffer before sample loading, use a 2.2-mL centrifuge tube. We found that if we used a 1.5-mL tube, the bottom of the column is sitting in the eluted buffer, thus leaving some buffer stuck in the bottom of the column. The 2.2-mL tube is big enough such that the column and buffer are separated.

12. It is not necessary to bring all the RNAs up to the same volume. We have found that hybridization appears to work well with hybridization buffer concentrations from 30–80%. Thus, differences in RNA volumes will not alter the hybridization.

13. We have obtained good results with as little as 100 ng of total RNA/reaction. Optimally, you should use 5 or 10 µg/reaction. You just need to test your system. Chemokines tend to be expressed more highly than most genes.

14. If RNA is very limiting, dissolve the RNA directly in 8–10 µL of hybridization buffer × number of probes you want to test. We have stored RNA at –70°C in this manner and it is fine.

15. Hybridization appears to be identical when between 0.5–1.5 million

cpm are added per reaction. We have even obtained good results with 100,000 cpm/reaction but we do try to maintain at least 500,000 cpm/reaction. You need to be in probe excess.

16. Once we forgot to turn the hybridization temperature from 90°C to 56°C for about 45 min. The assay still worked fine.

17. You can freeze the hybridization cocktail at –70°C after hybridization and RNase the next day if you use ^{33}P-UTP to label your probes.

18. Be sure to set up two control tubes containing probe and hybridization buffer and either just yeast tRNA or no RNA at all.

19. There is a lot of flexibility in time of RNase treatment. We have performed this for more than 1 h at 30°C with no problem.

20. We have compared RNase treatment at 30°C and 37°C and saw no difference.

21. Be sure to mix your glycoblue precipitate after you thaw it. If you look at it after thawing, you will see that some material has settled in the tube.

22. Shake the inactivation/precipitation solution vigorously right before you aliquot it. You need to make sure each tube gets the same amount of carrier RNA and glycoblue precipitate.

23. If you use the Proteinase K to inactivate the RNases, we found you can directly precipitate the protected RNA without phenol/chlorofom extraction.

24. We find using microfuge tubes of different colors to be extremely helpful. They are useful for grouping together RNAs in the appropriate experimental sets and also help you decide where to skip lanes in a gel for technical reasons (i.e., a bubble in the gel) or for publication purposes. We have never seen the color leach out of the tubes. We do autoclave the tubes in large glass beakers.

25. Do *not* siliconize the tubes that you use to pellet your protected RNA! If you do, the pellet will slide out of the tube when you decant the inactivation/precipitation solution. After we pour out the solution, we tap the tube rather hard on a Kimwipe tissue to remove liquid before we use the cotton swab. We have never lost a pellet by doing this although we see, on very rare occasions, the pellet migrate a little bit down the tube.

26. We do *not* change cotton swabs for each tube. We use one cotton swab/six tubes and have never transferred radioactivity from the swab to a tube. You do need to remove all excess liquid as possible as you want to load the entire sample in the well.

27. Regarding the decanting step, we put a piece of parafilm under the two layers of Kimwipes that we use to blot the liquid before using the cotton swab. This protects the bench pads from becoming contaminated with the isotope.

28. Resuspend every pellet in 3 µL of sample buffer by pipetting up and down (of course with a different pipet tip for each sample). Once we tried to resuspend the pellet by mixing with a vortex mixer and the gel turned out completely blank! While this may have been a coincidence, we do not subject the final sample to mixing this way.

29. You can also freeze the samples in the sample buffer at –70°C overnight. This only works with ^{33}P.

30. Load about 80,000–100,000 cpm in the probe-only lane. Resuspend the pellet in this tube to give you about 80,000–100,000 cpm/µL and use only 1 µL for the gel.

31. Put any excess inactivation/precipitation solution in a 1.5-mL microfuge tube and store it at –20°C with the rest of your reagents. This is very useful as we occasionally end up a little bit short when we are dispensing the 250 µL/tube. Just remember to mix it well before you use it.

32. Check with your radiation safety program to see if they want you to keep ^{33}P waste separate from other radioactive waste. Scintillation counters cannot distinguish between ^{33}P and ^{35}S and this may be a problem in your program.

33. A recipe for producing inactivation buffer as well as a co-precipitate solution was recently published *(8)*.

34. For a commercial gel mix, we use Invitrogen-Life Technologies Gel mix 6 Cat. no. 15543-010.

35. Make fresh ammonium persulfate every 2 wk.

36. Coat one plate with Sigmacote Sigma #SL-2.

37. Plates should be stripped every 7–10 gels, soak gel plates 20 min in 2 *N* NaOH.

38. When pouring plates, we usually elevate the plates by putting a pipet under the top part of gel plates and remove it after gel is poured. Allow gel to polymerize laying flat for about 20 min.

39. If you need quantitation, put gels on a scanner overnight (e.g., Molecular Dynamics Typhoon system) and then on film for 1–7 d. Otherwise go right on film. If you used 10 µg of total RNA per lane, you may only need a 4–6-h exposure for publication quality results. Obviously, the less RNA used, the longer you will need to expose

the film. The new intensifying screens and film designed for ^{33}P from Kodak are much more sensitive and permit shorter exposures.

40. Using the multiprobe template sets, you can quantitate your target gene relative to the L32 ribosomal RNA and/or GAPDH.

41. Are your films faint after overnight exposure and have a slightly cloudy background? Your developing solutions may be bad! I have found that at the very least, when using 1 µg of total RNA, the control genes should give a nice signal after overnight exposure.

42. If your darkroom has a computer in it, make sure the monitor is turned off before you open your film cassettes.

43. The new BioMax MS film from Kodak is ultra-sensitive. Not all safe-lights are truly "safe" for this film. If you are not sure, turn off the safelite when developing your film.

References

1. Schlievert, P. M. (1993) Role of superantigens in human disease. *J. Infect. Dis.* **167,** 997–1002.

2. Choi, Y., Kotzin, B., Hernon, L., Callahan, J., Marrack, P., and Kappler, J. (1989) Interaction of Staphylococcus aureus toxin "superantigens" with human T cells. *Proc. Natl. Acad. Sci. USA* **86,** 8941–8945.

3. Gascoigne, N. R. J. and Ames, K. T. (1991) Direct binding of secreted TCR β chain to superantigen associated with MHC class II complex protein. *Proc. Natl. Acad. Sci. USA* **88,** 613–616.

4. Kotzin, B. L., Leung, D. Y. M., Kappler, J., and Marrack, P. A. (1993) Superantigens and their potential role in human disease. *Adv. Immunol.* **54,** 99–166.

5. Krakauer, T. (1999) Immune response to staphylococcal superantigens. *Immunol. Res.* **20,** 163–173.

6. Jupin, C., Anderson, S., Damais, C., Alouf, J. E., and Parant, M. (1988) Toxic shock syndrome toxin 1 as an inducer of human tumor necrosis factors and gamma interferon. *J. Exp. Med.* **167,** 752–761.

7. Parsonnet, J., Hickman, R. K., Eardley, D. D., and Pier, G. B. (1985) Induction of human interleukin-1 by toxic shock syndrome toxin-1. *J. Infect. Dis.* **151,** 514–522.

8. Chesney, P. J., Davis, J. P., Purdy, W. K., Wand, P.J., and Chesney, R. W. (1981) Clinical manifestations of toxic shock syndrome. *J. Am. Med. Assoc.* **246,** 741–748.

9. Miethke, T., Wahl, C., Heeg, K., Echtenacher, B., Krammer, P. B., and Wagner, H. (1992) T cell-mediated lethal shock triggered in mice by the superantigen SEB: critical role of TNF. *J. Exp. Med.* **175,** 91–98.

10. Miethke, T., Wahl, C., Regele, D., Gaus, H., Heeg, K., and Wagner, H. (1993) Superantigen mediated shock: a cytokine release syndrome. *Immunbiology* **189,** 270–284.

11. Melton, D. A., Krieg, P. A., Rebagliati, M. R., Maniatis, T., Zinn, K., and Green, M. R. (1984) Efficient in vitro synthesis of biologically active RNA and RNA hybridization probes from plasmids containing a bacteriophage SP6 promoter. *Nucl. Acids Res.* **12,** 7035–7056.

12. Krupp, G. (1988) RNA synthesis: strategies for the use of bacteriophage RNA polymerases. *Gene* **72,** 75–89.

13. Okada, C. Y. and Weissman, I. L. (1989) Relative V beta transcript levels in thymus and peripheral lymphoid tissues from various mouse strains. Inverse correlation of I-E and Mls expression with relative abundance of several V beta transcripts in peripheral lymphoid tissues. *J. Exp. Med.* **169,** 1703–1719.

14. Kono, D. H., Baccala, R., Balderas, R. S., Kovac, S. J., Heald, P. W., Edelson, R. L., and Theofilopoulos, A. N. (1992) Application of a multiprobe RNase protection assay and junctional sequences to define V beta gene diversity in Sezary syndrome. *Am. J. Pathol.* **140,** 823–830.

15. Muller, K., Ehlers, S., Solbach, W., and Laskay, T. (2001) Novel multiprobe RNase protection assay (RPA) sets for the detection of murine chemokine gene expression. *J. Immunol. Methods* **249,** 155–165.

16. Luckow, B., Maier, H., Chilla, S., and Perez, de L. G. (2000) The mCK-5 multiprobe RNase protection assay kit can yield erroneous results for the murine chemokines IP-10 and MCP-1. *Anal. Biochem.* **286,** 193–197.

17. Hallensleben, W., Biro, L., Sauder, C., Hausmann, J., Asensio, V. C., Campbell, I. L., and Staeheli, P. A. (2000) Polymorphism in the mouse crg-2/IP-10 gene complicates chemokine gene expression analysis using a commercial ribonuclease protection assay. *J. Immunol. Methods* **234,** 149–151.

18. Harju, S. and Peterson, K. R. (2001) Sensitive ribonuclease protection assay employing glycogen as a carrier and a single inactivation/precipitation step. *Biotechniques* **30,** 1198–1204.

12

Staining Protocol for Superantigen-Induced Cytokine Production Studied at the Single-Cell Level

Lars Björk

1. Introduction

1.1. Everything Starts with the Quality of the Specimen

In order to get the full picture of the cytokine response generated by stimulation of various pathogens and superantigens in particular it is of crucial importance to collect data at various timepoints after stimulation. It is clear from those experiments performed that the production of the inflammatory and regulatory cytokines studied, differs in peak expression point and even cellular source depending on the time point studied *(1,2)*. One other aspect of the importance of kinetics is that when one studies the cytokine profile of a human derived specimen, e.g., peripheral blood mononuclear cells (PBMC) the response varies between different donors both in number of cytokines produced, level of production as well as the kinetic of the response.

1.2. Fixation and Permeabilization

To detect intracellular antigens such as cytokines the cells need to be made permeable for the detecting antibody. Permeabilization often requires a fixation step to stabilize the plasma membrane and

From: *Methods in Molecular Biology, vol. 214: Superantigen Protocols*
Edited by: T. Krakauer © Humana Press Inc., Totowa, NJ

block solubilization of the targeted proteins. The generation of a successful staining described in this chapter is primarily owing to the usage of the fixative formaldehyde, combined with the permeabilizer saponin and a careful selection of appropriate cytokine-specific antibodies.

1.3. The Current Protocol

The subheading of this section illustrates the constant changes of the intracellular staining method . The protocol described herein has mainly been developed in the laboratory of Professors Jan Andersson and Ulf Andersson at the Stockholm University since the mid-1980s *(3)* and has been reviewed previously by Sander et al. *(4)*. Although the technique was initially developed for immunofluorescence we have also adapted a protocol for immunoenzymatic staining. This has made it possible to perform intracellular staining of cytokines in tissue samples, which previously was troublesome due to the autofluorescence often present in tissue specimens *(5)*. In **Table 1** the major steps of the staining procedure are outlined.

1.4. Antibody Reagents

The antibodies described for cytokine staining are various mouse and rat monoclonals (listed in Materials). They have been selected by an extensive empirical evaluation of their signal to noise ratio and their capability to bind to an antigen that can withstand the fixation and permeabilization protocol. Most of the antibodies that have been tested have not given a desired staining quality and sometimes several hundred different clones have been tried before a proper and specific activity has been achieved. The antibodies listed here are the ones that we have to found work well with the combination of formaldehyde as a fixative and saponin as a permeabilizer.

1.5. Enumeration of Cytokine-Producing Cells

Our approach to cytokine assessment has been the use of an immunocytochemical technique to detect the intracellular presence

Table 1[a]
Steps for Staining Activated Cells for Intracellular Cytokines

1. Activation (Superantigen, LPS, PMA, etc.)
2. Harvest cells (on adhesion slides, *see* **Note 6**)
3. Fix with 4% PFA
4. Permeabilize and wash with saponin (0.1%)
5. Primary anti-cytokine antibody (diluted in 0.1% saponin)
6. Secondary fluorochrome conjugated antibody (diluted in 0.1% saponin)
7. Nuclear counter staining
8. Mount and record

[a]The current protocol used in the laboratory is described more thoroughly in **Subheading 3.**

of cytokines prior to secretion at the single cell level. A characteristic focal juxtanuclear staining-pattern reflecting the accumulation of the protein in the secretory ER-Golgi route has greatly facilitated the distinction between specific cytokine producers and cytokine binding cells (*see* **Figs. 1** and **2**; *see* **Note 1**). By developing an image analysis procedure for the enumeration of cytokine producing cells we have been able to appreciate these morphologic criteria. The system has allowed us to measure parameters of staining intensity as well as to assess the actual cell size in μm^2. The image analysis system is capable of discriminating cytokine producing cells from cytokine-binding cells *(6,7)*.

Similar results have, in our hands, been difficult to obtain by the use of flow cytometry. The reasons for these obstacles have been that the intensity of the fluorescent staining detecting the accumulated cytokine intracellulary and the autofluorescence from blast transformed cells sometimes overlap, or that the secreted cytokine has bound to its receptor and is present on the surface of target cells. However, today there has been a number of successful reports and protocol descriptions on flow cytometric analysis of cytokine-producing cells *(8–11)* combined with inhibitors of protein secretions, such as monensin *(9,11,12)* or brefeldin A *(13)* to increase the staining signal. Together with cell-sorting/gating or cell depletion this has proved to be a promising way to facilitate the assessment of

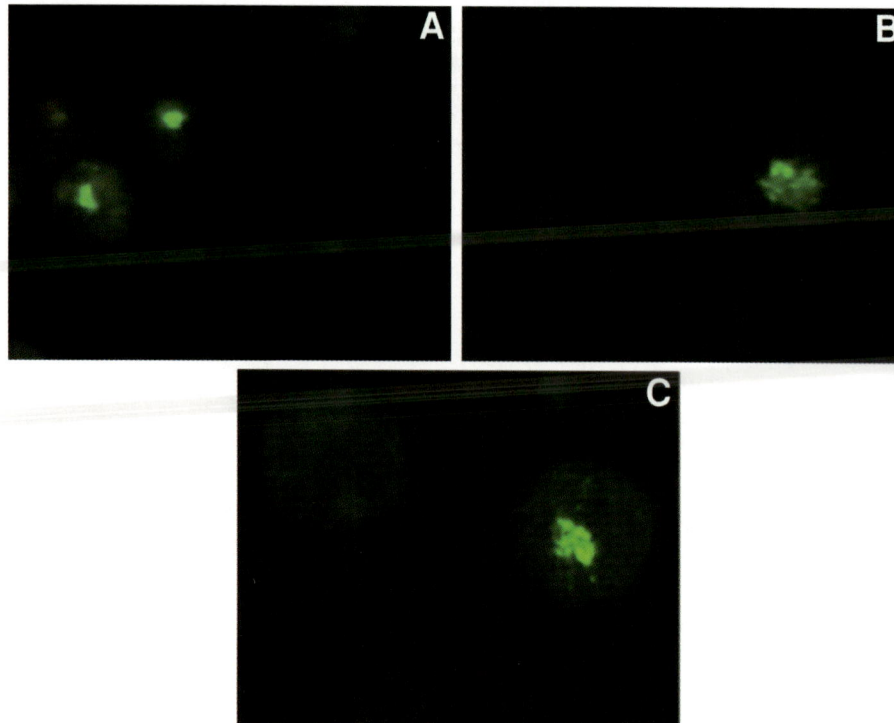

Fig. 1. Characteristics of intracellular cytokine staining pattern. (**A**) Cells producing IL-6 after 12 h of staphylococcal enterotoxn A (SEA). (**B**) Cells producing TNF-α after 4 h of SEA stimulation. (**C**) Cells producing IL-8 after 48 h of streptococcal pyrogenic exotoxin A (SPE-A) stimulation. Note the distinct juxtanuclear pattern reflecting the accumulation of the cytokine prior to secretion, which is evident in all of the micrographs.

cytokine producing cells in flow cytometry, especially in combination with the long wavelength fluorochromes that are now available. Today there are commercial suppliers of standardized kit with directly conjugated antibodies for cytokine analysis by flow cytometry. Further investigation is however required on the effects of the protein secretion inhibitors on cell activation and protein production. A capability but sometimes also a limitation of flow cytometry is the need for large sample number of cells in order to adjust and perform the analysis. In a clinical setting the frequency of cytokine producing cells are often low and when dealing with

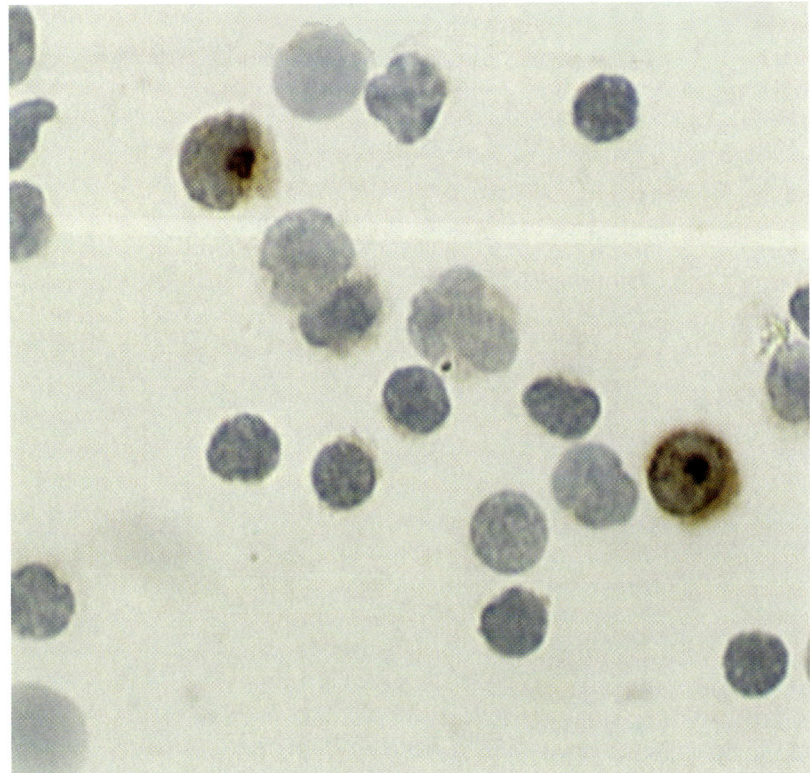

Fig. 2. Cytokine (IL-6) apperance in individual cells on adhesion slides after immunoenzymatic staining using DAB as substrate and counter-stained with hematoxilin.

human samples the actual total number of cells retrieved are often very low. Under these circumstances image analysis and the laser-scanner cytometer described below is probably the most effective tool for automated quantification of single cells (*see* **Table 2**).

Recently I have adapted an application for quantification of cytokine producing cells using the newly developed Laser Scan-ning Cytometer (LSC) from CompuCyte Corp. (Cambridge, MA). The LSC *(14)* (is a fluorescent scanner and enumerator just as a flow) cytometer but instead of a sheet fluid system the cells are scanned on a microscopic slide by the attached microscope and motorized stage (*see* **Fig. 3**). The LSC is thereby combining the

Table 2
Summary of the Features of Three Different Enumeration Systems Used for Cytokine Analysis

Flow cytometry	Image analysis	Laser-scanning cytometer
Rapid acquirement of multiple cells	No gating needed	No gating needed
Possibility to measure multiple events using fluorescent markers	Monitoring of the analysis	Monitoring of the analysis
Large sample numbers needed	Segmentation of doublets and triplets	Possible to detect small samples and low incidences
Need secretion inhibitors to enhance the signal	Possible to detect small samples and low incidences	Verification using re-examination procedure for positive cells
	Trouble in separation of double-labeled cells	Possibility to measure multiple events using fluorescent markers

generation of fluorescent histogram population data as in flow cytometry with the higher resolution and microscopic slide analysis capacity of an image analysis system.

Because the LSC is capable of measuring the overall intensity of the cell as well as the intracellular peak intensity, the same morphological criteria can be used to discriminate between positive cytokine producing cells and nonproducing cells. This feature of the LSC, called "probe analysis," removes the need for secretion inhibitors prior to harvesting since it is not the intensity per se, which is the discriminating parameter but the combination of the intensity and its intracellular localization. One additional feature, which is possible in image analysis and highly developed in the LSC system, is that the exact position of every cell scored on the microscopic slide can be registered and is put into as a part of the listmode file. This means that for example, when dealing with rare events, every single cell that has been scored positive by the system can be re-examined and a picture-gallery of the cells of interest can be generated (*see* **Fig. 4**).

1.6. Controls

The specificity of cytokine staining should be checked in parallel with isotype controls. Staining with the second step antibody alone and inhibition of the immunoreactivity by pre-absorption of the cytokine-specific antibody with relevant but not irrelevant cytokine are also relevant controls (*see* **Note 2**). Carefully chosen antibodies with tested specificity are used. One additional control, which is important when dealing with directly fluorochrome-conjugated antibodies, is to use a nonconjugated antibody to see whether the overall intensity of the staining is reduced.

The success of the intracellular staining techniques is primarily based on appreciation of staining morphology, which gives confidence in selecting positive cells even at low frequencies. In combination with kinetic analysis this will hopefully give a closer view of the full picture. In summary one can say that there is no golden standard for cytokine assessment. Multiple techniques must be used for opti-

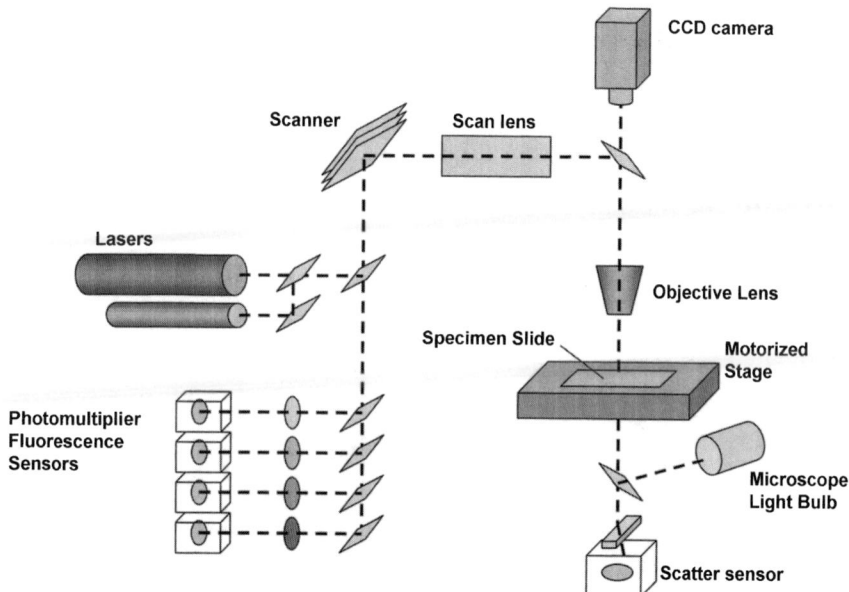

Fig. 3. Optical configuration of the Laser Scanner Cytometer.

mal information and it is of course the net effect of secreted agonists, antagonists, and agonists adsorbed by soluble and cell-surface decoy receptors that determines the biological signal of cytokines.

2. Materials

2.1. Buffers

1. Fixation Buffer: Four gram paraformaldehyde (PFA) (Sigma, St. Louis, MO) is dissolved in 10 mL double-distilled water. The mixture is heated to 70°C for 2 h and a few drops of 2 *M* NaOH are added until the solution becomes clear. 0.54 gram glucose is added. The 40% formaldehyde solution is diluted to 4% with PBS and the pH is adjusted to 7.4. Cool down to +4°C (*see* **Note 3**).
2. Washing buffer: Earls Buffered Salt Solution (EBSS) (Gibco-BRL, Paisly, UK). Adjust pH to 7.4–7.6.
3. Washing buffer with saponin: EBSS (Gibco-BRL, Paisly, UK) with 0.1% (w/v) saponin (Riedel de Haen, Seelze, Germany). Adjust pH to 7.4–37.6. (*see* **Note 4**).

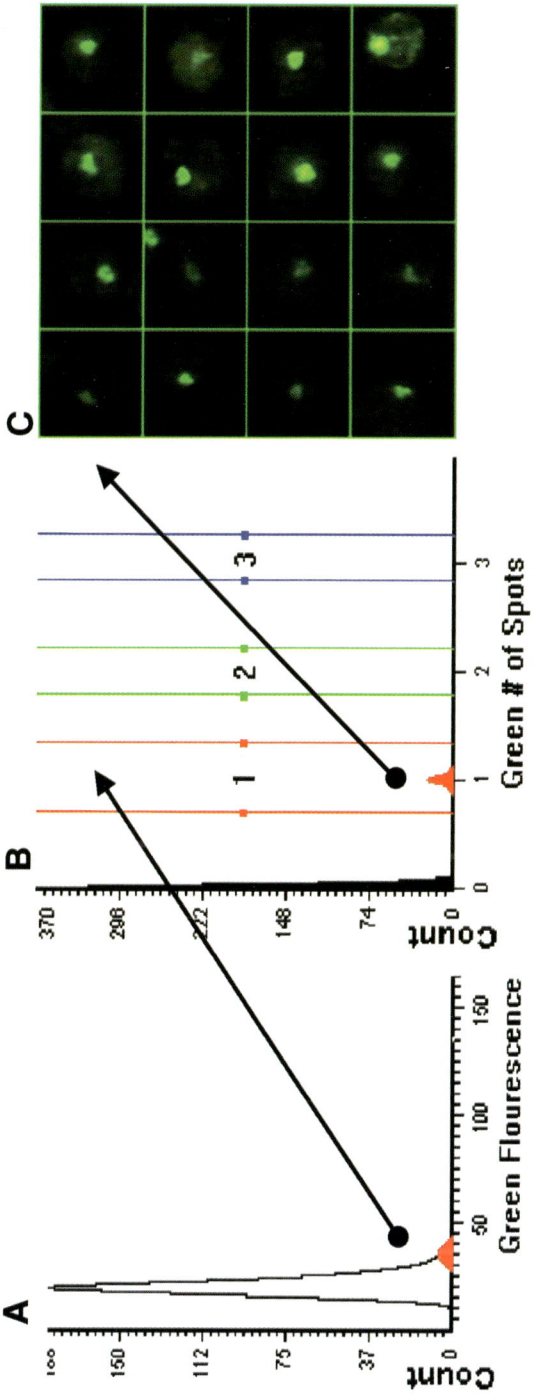

173

Fig. 4. The Laser Scanning Cytometer can score the cytokine positive cells based on the morphology and peak intensity of the cytokine staining. Note that the overall intensity of the cytokine positive cells are not sufficient to get a clear shift in the two populations when secretion inhibitors are not used (A). The positive cells, with a distinct intracellular peak is detected by the intracellular spot counting capability of the LSC (B). The re-examination protocol (CompuSort™) of the LSC show a gallery of cells in gate 1 of the B histogram (C).

4. Peroxidase Blocking Buffer: 0.3 M NaN$_3$ and 1% H$_2$O$_2$ with 0.1% (w/v) saponin.
5. Avidin Biotin Blocking Kit: Commercial kit from Vector Lab. (Burlingame, CA) supplemented with 0.1% (w/v) saponin.
6. Vectastain Avidin Biotin Complex (ABC) kit: Commercial kit from Vector Lab. (Burlingame, CA) supplemented with 0.1% (w/v) saponin.
7. Nuclear counter-staining solution for fluorescent assay with LSC: EBSS with RNAse (QIAGEN, Hamburg, Germany/propidium iodide (PI) (Sigma, St. Louis, MO) (200 µg/mL/50 µg/mL).
8. Nuclear counter-staining solution for immunoenzymatic staining: Mayer's Hematoxilin Counterstain (Sigma, St. Louis, MO).
9. Anti-fade mounting solution: Slow Fade Light (Molecular Probes, Eugene, OR) (*see* **Note 5**).
10. Immunoenzymatic mounting solution: PBS and glycerol 1:9 (v/v).

2.2. Reagents

1. Antibodies: Please *see* **Tables 3** and **4**.
2. Horseradish Peroxidase (HRP) substrates for immunoenzymatic staining:
   a. DAB, ABC kit (Vector Laboratories).
   b. AEC (Sigma).
   c. 4CN (Vector Laboratories).

2.3. Equipment

1. Microscopic slides: 12-well Adhesion Slides (Superior, Lauda-Köningshofen, Germany) (*see* **Note 6**).
2. Humid incubation chamber: Typically a large petri dish with light protective cover and a wet cellulose tissue.
3. Quantitative Image Analysis equipment: A Leica DMRDA microscope hooked up to a Quantimet 550 IW image analysis system (Leica Microsystem, Cambridge, UK) equipped with a CCD 24-bit color camera (Hamamatsu, Japan). A dedicated high-level software routine was written in order to get the automated flow of morphometric and densitometric analysis of the cytokine-producing cells *(6)*.
4. Laser-Scanning Cytometer: LSC equipped with two laser system Argon 488nm and HeNe 633nm and four PMT from Compucyte Corp. (Cambridge, MA).

3. Method

3.1. Cytokine Detection at the Single Cell Level Using Immunofluorescent Staining Technique

1. Harvest the cultured cells and wash in cold, serum-free washing buffer (EBSS) by approx 3 repeated centrifugations. The cells need to be washed free of proteins in order to adhere properly to the adhesion slides. Be careful to dispose the first supernatant in biological toxic waste due to presence of superantigens.

2. The protective film of the reaction fields of the adhesion slide are washed away. After this step the slide should have a drop of buffer on the wells and be kept in a humidified chamber throughout the staining procedure, especially before fixation of the cells in order to prevent cell loss. Transfer 10 µL of cell suspension ($1–5 \times 10^6$ cells/mL) to the wells of the adhesion slide and allow them to adhere for 10 min at room temperature (*see* **Note 6** regarding adhesion slides).

3. Wash away unbound cells with washing buffer. When washing the adhesion slides it is convenient to add one drop per well of the slide and flip that drop away by a wrist movement. If one use a slide-cuvet make sure to have appropriate amount of buffer to get proper washing conditions. Suction is not recommended since it often causes too much cell loss.

4. Fix the adhered cells with cold formaldehyde in darkness for 10 min.

5. Wash away formaldehyde and unbound cells three times with EBSS washing buffer.

6. To block the reaction fields on the adhesion slides and any remaining activity of the formaldehyde with 2% fetal bovine serum (FBS) diluted in EBSS washing buffer. Incubate for 5 min in 37°C.

7. Wash the fixed cells three times with washing buffer containing 0.1% saponin. Wipe carefully between the wells with a filter paper to ensure that the wells are not connected with a "water-bridge." IMPORTANT NOTE: Saponin should now be present throughout the staining procedure (*see* **Note 4**).

8. Incubate with cytokine-specific antibody (2–10 µg/mL) diluted in EBSS-saponin supplemented with 0.02% NaN$_3$, for 30 min at room temperature. Approximately 10 µL is enough to cover one well on the adhesion slide.

9. Wash the cells three times with washing buffer containing 0.1% saponin. Wipe carefully between the wells with a filter paper to

Table 3
Antibodies Suitable for Cytokine Detection in Human Cells[a]

Cytokine	Antibody	Isotype	Source	References
IL-1α	1277-89-7	mouse (m)IgG1	Immunokontact, Switzerland	(15; see **Note 1**)
	1277-82-23	mIgG1	Immunokontact, Switzerland	(15; see **Note 1**)
	1279-143-4	mIgG1	Immunokontact, Switzerland	(15; see **Note 1**)
IL-1β	2D8	mIgG1	Immunokontact, Switzerland	(15; see **Note 1**)
IL-1ra	1384-92-17-19	mIgG1	Immunokontact, Switzerland	(15)
IL-2	MQ1-17H12	rat(r) IgG2a	Pharmingen, CA	(16)
	BG-5	mIgG1	Serotec, UK	
IL-3	BVD8-6G8	rIgG	Pharmingen, CA	(16)
	BVD3-IF9	rIgG1	DNAX, CA	(16)
IL-4	MP4-25D2	rIgG1	Pharmingen, CA	(16)
IL-5	JES-39D10	rIgG2a	Pharmingen, CA	(16)
IL-6	MQ2-6A3	rIgG	DNAX, CA	(16)
	IG61	mIgG1	Toray Ltd, Japan	(17)
IL-8	NAP-1	mIgG1	Sandoz	(18)

IL-10	JES3-19F1	rIgG2a	DNAX, CA	(16)
	JES3-12G8	rIgG2a	Pharmingen, CA	(16)
IL-13	JES8-5A2	rIgG2a	Biosource Int. USA	
	JES8-30F11	rIgG2a	DNAX, CA	
GM-CSF	BVD2-21C11	rIgG2a	Pharmingen, CA	(16)
	BVD2-5A2	rIgG2a	Pharmingen, CA	(16)
G-CSF	BVD13-3A5	rIgG	DNAX, CA	
G-CSF	BVD11-37G10	rIgG	DNAX, CA	
TNF-α	MAB1	mIgG1	Pharmingen, CA	
TNF-α	MAB11	mIgG1	Pharmingen, CA	(6)
	MP9-20A4	rIgG	DNAX, CA	(16)
TNF-β	LTX21	mIgG2b	Biosource Int, USA	(19)
TNF-β	LTX22	mIgG1	Bender MedSystems, Austria	(19)
IFN-γ	D1K1	mIgG1	Mabtech, Stockholm, Sweden	(20)
IFN-γ	7-B-6	mIgG1	Mabtech, Stockholm, Sweden	(20)

[a]The primary antibodies are diluted to approx 2–10 µg/mL in washing buffer with saponin and supplemented with 0.02% NaN$_3$. Undiluted stock antibodies are kept sterile in +4°C or aliquoted into small samples stored in −70°C. Repeated freeze and thaw cycles are not recommended.

Table 4
Secondary Reagents Suitable for Cytokine Detection in Single Cells

Antibody	Dilution	Species	Conjugate	Source
Anti-mouse IgG1	1:300	Goat	Biotin	Caltag Laboratories, CA
Anti-mouse IgG1	1:300	Goat	FITC	Caltag Laboratories, CA
Anti-mouse IgG2	1:300	Goat	Biotin	Caltag Laboratories, CA
Anti-mouse IgG2	1:300	Goat	FITC	Caltag Laboratories, CA
Anti-rat Ig	1:300	Goat	Biotin	Vector Laboratories, CA
Anti-rat Ig	1:300	Goat	FITC	Vector Laboratories, CA
Anti-mouse IgG	1:200	Goat	Alexa 488	Molecular Probes, OR
Streptavidin	1:200		Alexa 488	Molecular Probes, OR
Vectastain EliteAccording to manufacturers protocolVector Laboratories, CA				

ensure that the wells are not connected with a "water-bridge."

10. Incubate with appropriate fluorochrome-conjugated secondary reagent for 30 min at room temperature, diluted in EBSS with saponin. Include 5% human AB serum to reduce background problem with the polyclonal antisera. Incubate in darkness (10 μL antibody solution/well on a 12-well adhesion slide).

In order to further amplify the fluorescent signal one can also use biotinylated antibodies in this step and after washing add an extra incubation step with fluorochrome-conjugated streptavidin.

11. Wash the cells three times with washing buffer containing 0.1% saponin.

12. Wash the cells with washing buffer EBBS without saponin.

13. If counterstaining is desired which is required for LSC analysis or DNA index analysis, incubate with nuclear counterstaining buffer containing propidium iodide and RNAse for 30 min at room temperature.

14. Wash the cells with washing buffer EBBS without saponin, leave the cells to dry out slightly and mount the slide in antifading mounting media (*see* **Note 5**).

3.2. Cytokine Detection at the Single-Cell Level Using Immunoenzymatic Staining Technique

1. Harvest and fixation of cultured cells on the adhesion slide for enzymatic staining is identical to the previously described method in **Subheadings 3.1., steps 1–6**.

2. Block endogenous peroxidase activity with Peroxidase Blocking Buffer for 30 min at room temperature.

3. Wash the fixed cells with washing buffer with 0.1% saponin as described in **Subheading 3.1., step 7**.

4. First step incubation with anti-cytokine antibody is performed identical to **Subheading 3.1., step 8**.

5. Wash the cells three times with washing buffer with 0.1% saponin as described in **Subheading 3.1., step 9**.

6. Incubate with appropriate biotinylated secondary reagent for 30 min in room temperature, diluted in EBSS with saponin and 5% human AB serum to reduce background problem with the polyclonal antisera (10 μL antibody solution/well on a 12-well adhesion slide).

7. Wash the cells three times with washing buffer with 0.1% saponin.

8. Incubate with pre-diluted Vectastain ABC diluted in washing buffer with 0.1% saponin for 30 min at room temperature and darkness.
9. Wash the cells with washing buffer EBBS without saponin. Wipe between the wells with a filter paper.
10. Prepare appropriate substrate according to the protocol given by the manufacturer. Substrate should always be freshly made. The color reaction is developed at room temperature and darkness for approx 8 min. The reaction is stopped with washing buffer without saponin.
11. If counterstaining is desired, incubate with hematoxilin for 1–10 s and rinse in washing buffer without saponin.
12. Mount the slide in immunoenzymatic mounting solution.

4. Notes

When performing staining that is to be enumerated by an automated cytometry unit, either a flow cytometer, image analysis equipment or the laser scanning cytometer, careful considerations has to be taken for all the steps, from harvesting and fixation to mounting solution and high quality cover slip, so that the general conditions including temperatures, incubation times and working solutions are the same for a given experiment.

1. Certain members of the interleukin-1 (IL-1) family lacks the signal sequence and hence are not secreted through the classical secretory pathway. The staining morphology of these cytokines is sometimes spread throughout the cytoplasm in a filamentous pattern resembling that of the cytoskeleton *(15)*. Attaching the signal sequence from the IL-1receptor antagonist can indeed modulate the staining pattern of IL-1β. In mouse fibroblasts (NIH3T3) transfected with this signal sequence-IL-1β construct, cells exhibited a Golgi-localized staining pattern *(21)*. This strongly supports the role for the signal peptide sequence in the generation of the observed intracellular staining morphology.
2. To check the specificity of the anti-cytokine antibody we generally perform a co-incubation at +4°C overnight with the detecting antibody and recombinant cytokine at a 1:10 molar ratio prior to staining. The overnight incubation is done in washing buffer without saponin and saponin is then added prior to staining of the specimen.
3. In long-term storage, formaldehyde deteriorates into methanol and formic acid and hence the working solution is preferably used freshly

diluted. Short-term storage (few hours) can be done at +4°C protected from light. Formaldehyde should be used in fume hoods due to its allergenic and toxic properties. One can also prepare formaldehyde from 37% formalin and dilute it to 2%. Make sure to check the pH to 7.4 for optimal results.

4. The use of saponin as permeabilizers in order to allow the anticytokine antibodies to penetrate into the prefixed cells has, in our hands, shown to be the most advantageous of all tested detergents, permeabilizers and organic solvents used to facilitate detection of intracellular antigens including: Triton X-100, n-octyl-beta-D-glycopyranoside, acetone, methanol and ethanol. Saponin is a generic name for a family of glycosides derived from plants. Saponin exists in several plant species but the saponin used in this study is derived from the South American tree Quillaja saponaria. It has been suggested that the mechanism of permeabilization with saponin is an intercalation of saponins in the membrane *(22)* and that this is a reversible process. Supporting this notion is the fact that a pretreatment with saponin is not sufficient to render the cells permeable for antibodies, and saponin need to be constantly present when incubating with an intracellular targeted antibody *(4,22,23)*.

5. Although the commercial antifading solution from Molecular Probes is excellent, especially when using their Alexa-dye conjugates, we have also been successful with the following antifading solution: Carbonate/Bicarbonate buffered glycerol (1:1 v/v) containing 2% (w/v) 1.4 diazabicyclo [2,2,2] octane (Sigma) and adjust pH to 7.4. When mounting a microscopic slide take care to get an even distribution of the mounting media and as thin as possible in order to get the best optical quality of your specimen.

6. The 12-well adhesion slides (*see* **Fig. 5**) with commercial quality poly L-lysin coating and a hydrophobic ring are excellent harvesting slides which minimizes the required amount of sampled cells and reagents as well as reducing the risk of cross-contamination between wells. No selection for certain members of living cells of the peripheral blood mononuclear cell (PBMC) preparation has been shown *(24)* and dead cells do not adhere to the adhesion slides. They are however sometimes difficult to get hold of in the US. They were previously sold by BIORAD Germany, but are now available directly from the manufacturer (Superior/Marienfeld Laboratory Glassware, Lauda-Köningshofen, Germany) (http://www.superior.de). Other electrostatic slides on the market are sometimes equally applicable

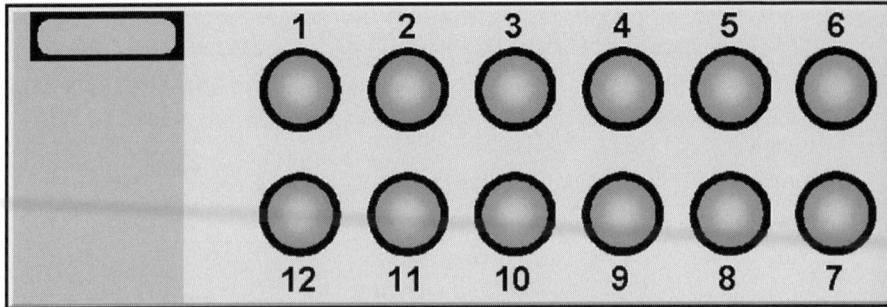

Fig. 5. The 12-well adhesion slide

depending on cell type used. Our personal experience is that it is quite easy to find slides which are effective in harvesting primary cells whereas continuous cell lines are more difficult to harvest on adhesion slides. Proper care need to be taken so that not all your samples are lost during harvesting and fixation. If adhesion slides are not applicable to your samples, one can also perform the staining steps in small centrifuge tubes and mount the cells on a traditional microscopic specimen slide prior to examination. Usually after fixation the cells are firmly adhered to the slides and can withstand repeated washing steps and incubations. If the cells are left to dry after fixation one can also store them for long periods (several months) in dry conditions at −20°C without deterioration.

References

1. Björk, L., Andersson, J., Ceska M., and Andersson U. (1992) Endotoxin and Staphylococcus aureus enterotoxin a induced different patterns of cytokines. *Cytokine* **4,** 513–519.
2. Andersson, J., Nagy, S., Björk, L., Abrams, J., Holm, S., and Andersson U. (1992) Bacterial toxin induced cytokine production studied at the single cell level. *Immunol. Rev.* **127,** 69–96.
3. Andersson, U., Laskay, T., Andersson J., and DeLey, M. (1986) Phenotypic characterization of single gamma-interferon producing cells after OKT3 antibody activation. *Eur. J. Immunol.* **16,** 1457–1460.
4. Sander, B., Andersson, J., and Andersson, U. (1991) Assessment of cytokines by immuno.fluorescence and the paraformaldehyde/saponin procedure. *Immunol. Rev.* **119,** 65–93.
5. Andersson, J., Abrams, J., Björk, L., Funa, K., Litton, M., Ågren, K.,

and Andersson, U. (1994) Concomitant in vivo production of 19 different cytokines in human tonsils. *Immunology* **83,** 16–24.

6. Björk, L., Fehniger, T. E., Andersson, U., and Andersson, J. (1996) Computerised assessment of production of multiple human cytokines at the single cell level using image analysis. *J. Leukocyte Biol.* **59,** 287–295.

7. Björk, L., Andersson, U., Chauvet, J.-M, Skansén-Saphir U., and Andersson J. (1994) Quantification of superantigen induced IFN-γ production by computerised image analysis: inhibition of cytokine production and blast transformation by pooled human IgG. *J. Immunol. Methods* **175,** 201–213.

8. Assenmacher, M., Schmitz, J., and Radbruch, A. (1994) Flow cytometric determination of cytokines in activated murine T helper lymphocytes: expression of interleukin-10 and interferon-γ and interleukin-4 expressing cells. *Eur. J. Immunol.* **24,** 1097–1101.

9. Jung, T., Schauer, U., Heusser, C., Neumann, C., and Rieger, C. (1993) Detection of intracellular cytokines by flow cytometry. *J. Immunol. Methods* **159,** 197–207.

10. Ferrick, D. A., Schrenzel, M. D., Mulvania, T., Hsieh, B., Ferlin, W. G., and Lepper, H. (1995) Differential production of interferon-γ and interleukin-4 in response to Th1- and Th2-stimulating pathogens by γδ T cells in vivo. *Nature* **373,** 255–257.

11. Prussin, C. and Metcalf, D. D. (1995) Detection of intracytoplasmic cytokine using flow cytometry and directly conjugated anti-cytokine antibodies. *J. Immunol. Methods* **188,** 117–128.

12. Henter, J.-I., Söder, O., and Andersson, U. (1988) Identification of individual tumor necrosis factor/cachectin-producing cells after lipopolysaccharide induction. *Eur. J. Immunol.* **18,** 983–988.

13. Openshaw, P., Murphy, E. E., Hosken, N. A., Maino, V., Davis, K., Murphy, K., and O'Garra, A. (1995) Heterogeneity of intracellular cytokine synthesis at the single cell level in polarized T helper 1 and T helper 2 populations. *J. Exp. Med.* **182,** 1357–1367.

14. Kamentski, L. A., Burger, D. E., Gersham, R. J., Kamentski, L. D., and Luther, E. (1997) Slide-based laser scanning cytometry. *Acta. Cytol.* **41,** 123–143.

15. Andersson, J., Björk, L., Dinarello, C. A., and Andersson U. (1992) Lipopolysacharide induces human interleukin-1 receptor antagonist and interleukin-1 in the same cell. *Eur. J. Immunol.* **22,** 2617–2623.

16. Abrams, J. S., Roncarolo, H. G., Yssel, H., Andersson, U., Gleich, G. L., and Silver, J. E. (1992) Strategies of anti-cytokine monoclonal

antibody development:Immonuassay of IL-10 and IL-5 in clinical samples. *Immunol Rev.* **127,** 5–24.

17. Ida, N. (1989) Establishment of strongly neautralizing mAb to human IL-6 and its epitope analysis. *Biochem. Biophys. Res. Com.* **165,** 728–734.

18. Martich, G. D., Danner, R. L., Ceska, M., and Suffredini, A. F. (1991) Detection of IL-8 and TNF in normal humans after intravenous endotoxin. *J. Exp. Med.* **173,** 1021–1024.

19. Lamche, H. R. and Adolf, G. R. (1990) Highly sensitive immunoassay for antibodies to human tumor necrosis factor and lymphotoxin. *J. Immunol. Methods* **131,** 283–289.

20. Andersson, G., Ekre, H.-P., Alm, G., and Perlmann, P. (1989) Monoclonal antibody two-site ELISA for human IFN-γ. *J. Immunol. Methods* **25,** 89–96.

21. Gjörloff Wingren, A., Björkdahl, O., Labuda, T., Björk, L., Andersson, U., Gullberg, U., et al. (1996) Fusion of Signal Sequence to the Interleukin-1β gene directs the protein from cytoplasmatic accumulation to extracellular release. *Cell. Immunol.* **169,** 226–237.

22. Willingham, M. C. and Pastan, I. (1985) *An Atlas of Immunofluorescence in Cultured Cells.* Academic Press Inc., London, UK, pp. 2–11.

23. Willingham, M. C. (1980) Electron microscopic immunocytochemical localization of intracellular antigens in cultured cells: the EGS and ferritin bridge procedures. *Histochem. J.* **12,** 419–434.

24. Schneider, H., Vogt, A., and Bross, K. (1984) Identification of proliferating subpopulations in microcultures by surface marker and autoradiography. *Immunol. Commun.* **13,** 553–561.

13

Assessment of Specific T-Cell Activation by Superantigens

Natalie Sutkowski and Brigitte T. Huber

1. Introduction

The main characteristic of a superantigen (SAg) is that it activates specific subsets of T cells that are composed of particular T-cell receptor (TCR) variable region β chain gene products (TCRBV). SAgs are thought to form a bridge between the TCRBV region on the T cell and the MHC class II molecule on the antigen-presenting cell (APC). This bridging transduces a strong signal to the T cell through the TCR, resulting in T-cell activation, which is manifested by upregulation of cell-surface markers associated with activation, T-cell proliferation, and cytokine release. In this chapter we shall outline two methods for assessing specific T-cell activation based on the preceding criteria: 1) detection of markers of activation in individual TCRBV subsets early after SAg stimulation; and 2) analysis of cytokine release from TCRBV specific T-cell hybridomas in response to SAg presentation.

1.1. Bacterial vs Viral SAgs

SAgs are derived from two different types of pathogens: bacteria and viruses *(1)*. The bacterial SAgs are toxins, which are secreted

From: *Methods in Molecular Biology, vol. 214: Superantigen Protocols*
Edited by: T. Krakauer © Humana Press Inc., Totowa, NJ

proteins that can be purified and added directly to cultured cells at known concentrations. Hence, it is a relatively straightforward matter to stimulate T cells using bacterial toxins, and we would suggest that researchers planning to use the following methods, would initially test their hands with some of the common bacterial SAgs, such as staphylococcal enterotoxins (SEs) or toxic shock syndrome toxin (TSST). On the other hand, it is extremely difficult to purify the best-known viral SAg, mouse mammary tumor virus Mls; thus, to assess functional T-cell responses elicited by viral SAgs, it is necessary to use APC that express the SAg. These APC can be generated by transfecting the gene encoding the SAg into MHC class II^+ cell lines. Alternatively, there exist APC that express endogenous SAgs. A potential difficulty can arise in identifying APC that express the viral SAg, because Mls is expressed at very low levels in cells, and available antibodies are often incapable of detecting the protein either by Western-blotting technique or flow cytometry. Therefore, the recommended strategy for detecting Mls expression is to first assess transcriptional activation, and then look for functional activation of TCRBV specific T cells. This requires that the method chosen for identifying TCRBV specificity should be tried and tested prior to beginning such studies. Positive controls are essential, such as APC lines known to stably express the SAg, or bacterial SAgs with similar specificity.

1.2 Assessing Early T-Cell Activation with CD69

One method for detecting activation of primary TCRBV specific T cells, is to look for preferential expression of markers of activation on individual TCRBV subsets. An advantage to this method is that it can be completed in a single day if the marker of activation is expressed very early after T-cell signaling, such as CD69 (2). In addition, because CD69 is expressed prior to the production of cytokines, there is no cytokine activation of bystander T cells, which can obscure the results. A disadvantage of this method is that the anti-TCRBV antibodies, used to distinguish between individual TCRBV subsets are expensive, and antibodies are not currently available for all of the human TCRBV gene products.

CD69 can be expressed on lymphocytes as early as 1 h after activation, depending upon the stimulus. We have found that phorbol myristate acetate (PMA) causes a very rapid and strong induction of CD69 on peripheral blood cells, with virtually all of the cells expressing the marker at a high level within 1 h of treatment, as assessed by flow cytometry. On the other hand, the T cell mitogen phytohemagglutinin (PHA) causes activation of CD69 on approximately half of all T cells within 4–6 h after treatment. When assessing the expression of CD69 in individual TCRBV subsets, one finds that the marker is expressed equally in each subset after PHA stimulation *(3)*. This is exactly what would be expected from mitogen activation of T cells, where there is no TCRBV specificity. In contrast, if T cells are activated with the bacterial SAg SEB, stark differences in CD69 expression are seen between individual TCRBV subsets *(3)*. With human T cells, the highest expression of CD69 is on the TCRBV12 subset *(3)*. This correlates well with results derived from in vivo studies, in which the TCRBV12 subset is preferentially expanded after injection of SEB into SCID mice reconstituted with human lymphocytes *(4)*. CD69 has been used for identification of TCRBV specificity in response to the EBV associated SAg, HERV-K18 Env *(3)*; and to Mls *(5)*. In this system, where primary T cells are used, it is essential that autologous APC are used for SAg presentation.

1.3. Activation of TCRBV Specific T-Cell Hybridomas

A standard method for detection of SAg mediated T-cell responses is to assess activation of TCRBV specific T-cell hybridomas. T-cell hybridomas are generated by fusing primary T cells expressing particular *TCR* genes, with T-cell lymphomas *(6,7)*. Both mouse and human T-cell hybridomas exist. In addition, chimeric T-cell hybridomas have been generated by transfecting recombinant TCR-β chain gene constructs, consisting of human BV genes fused to murine β-chain diversity, join and constant region segments, into murine T-cell hybridomas lacking *BV* genes *(8)*. These chimeric hybridomas express the human *TCRBV* genes in isolation, in the context of murine CD3 and TCR-α chain; they were designed specifically for detecting human TCR binding to SAgs *(8)*. When T-cell hybridomas are activated, they secrete cytokines, usually IL-2, which can be measured in the cell supernatant either by enzyme-linked immunosorbent assay (ELISA) or by bioassay, i.e., measuring proliferation of a cytokine-dependent cell line *(9)*. SAg activation of TCRBV specific T-cell hybridomas can, therefore, be tested by measuring cytokine production.

This is a well-accepted means for establishing TCRBV restriction of a particular SAg. An advantage of this technique is that T-cell hybridomas do not require HLA-matched APC for SAg presentation, and therefore allogeneic or xenogeneic APC can be used to present the SAg *(8)*. In addition, costimulation during SAg presentation is not required. A disadvantage is that T-cell hybridomas are inherently unstable, and frequently lose surface CD3 spontaneously with in vitro culture, rendering them inactive. This can be overcome by limiting the length of time the hybrids are maintained in vitro, and also by frequent sorting of the hybrids for cells that stain CD3 bright.

2. Materials

2.1. CD69 Assay

1. Responders: Fresh human peripheral blood mononuclear cells (PBMC) isolated by ficoll gradient separation. Murine lymph-node cell or spleen-cell suspensions, red blood cells lysed with ammonium chloride solution, e.g., StemCell Technologies (Vancouver, Canada) or BD Pharmingen.
2. APC: For presentation of bacterial SAgs, there are sufficient APC present in PBMC or spleen cells, thus, it is unnecessary to add more. For presentation of viral SAgs, use autologous or MHC identical APC that express the viral SAg. Allogeneic or xenogeneic APC will greatly increase the background in this assay, obscuring results. APC can be generated by transfecting the viral SAg into a haploidentical MHC class II positive cell line.
3. 10% complete RPMI media: RPMI supplemented with 10% fetal calf serum (FCS), glutamine, Na pyruvate, HEPES, β-Mercaptoethanol, penicillin, streptomycin (Gibco-BRL). Use Dulbecco's PBS for washing cells.

4. Plastic ware: 6-well tissue culture plates, 96-well V-bottom plates, and FACS tubes.

5. Mitogens: Phytohemagglutinin (PHA), use at 2 μg/mL for human T cells. Concanavalin A (conA), use at 4 μg/mL for murine T cells. Stock solutions are prepared by dissolving PHA or conA, previously sterilized by UV or gamma irradiation, in PBS at a concentration of 1 mg/mL. Aliquots are stored frozen at –20°C. Both PHA and conA are available from Sigma.

6. Bacterial SAgs: SEA, SEB, SEC, SED, SEE, TSST-1, use at 0.1–1 mg/mL for murine and human T cells. Stock solutions are prepared by dissolving toxins, previously sterilized by UV or gamma irradiation, in PBS at a concentration of 1 mg/mL. Aliquots are stored frozen at –20°C. SEA, SEB, and TSST-1 are available from Sigma. A comprehensive list of highly purified toxins is available through Toxin Technology (Sarasota, FL). **Use safety precautions when working with toxins, e.g., wear gloves and/or masks, since they are very toxic even in minute doses.**

7. Viral SAgs: Use autologous or MHC identical APC expressing the viral SAgs. The dose is determined by varying the ratio of SAg-expressing APC to responding T cells (APC:responder ratio).

8. Anti-CD69 MAb, phycoerythrin (PE) or fluorescein isothiocyanate (FITC) conjugated, (BD Pharmingen).

9. Anti-TCRBV MAbs. BD Pharmingen sells a complete screening panel of FITC labeled anti-murine TCRBV MAbs, and individual anti-mouse TCRBV MAbs, purified or labeled with various fluorochromes. Anti-human TCRBV MAbs are sold by BD Pharmingen and Coulter Immunotech. Second stage reagent: FITC- or PE-labeled rabbit or goat anti-mouse Ig (Zymed).

10. FACS buffer. Ice cold Dulbecco's PBS supplemented with 2% FCS and 0.1% sodium azide. **Use safety precautions when working with sodium azide, e.g., wear gloves and/or masks; the powder form is very toxic when inhaled.**

11. Cell fixative. 1% paraformaldehyde in FACS buffer. 4% paraformaldehyde stock solution is prepared by dissolving 20 g paraformaldehyde (Sigma) in 500 mL Dulbecco's PBS, heat in 56°C water bath in fume hood until dissolved; pH to 7.5. Store at 4°C in dark. Dilute to 1% immediately prior to use.

12. Equipment. Tissue culture hoods, incubators (37°C, 5% CO_2), centrifuge, pipetmen.

13. Flow cytometry immunofluorescence analysis instruments, e.g., FACScan, or FACSCalibur by Becton Dickinson.

2.2. T-Cell Hybridoma Assay

1. TCRBV specific T-cell hybridomas. (Some available from ATCC). Expand in recommended media.
2. APC lines. (Many available from ATCC). For SAg presentation, the only absolute requirement for an APC is MHC class II. It is not necessary to use MHC-identical APC for activation of T-cell hybridomas; thus, allogeneic or xenogeneic APC lines may be used. Costimulatory molecules are not required, but may increase hybridoma responses. Examples of good APC are human and mouse B- lymphoma cell lines; macrophage cell lines; Epstein-Barr virus transformed human B-lymphoblastoid cell lines (LCL); fibroblast lines transfected with MHC class II, such as DAP cells *(10)*; Chinese hamster ovary (CHO) cells transfected with MHC class II, such as CHIE cells *(11)*. APC lines should be adapted for growth in media preferred for the T-cell hybridomas.
3. Media: Use media recommended by ATCC for hybridoma growth, **mycoplasma-free**. Test all media reagents consistently for mycoplasma. 0.2 μ filter all media reagents including FCS.
4. Freezer media: 90% fetal calf serum (FCS) and 10% DMSO.
5. Cell sorting MAbs. Anti-mouse CD3 MAb, clone 145 2C11; anti-mouse CD4 MAb, clone LT34; anti-human CD3 MAb, clone OKT3; anti-human CD4 MAb, clone OKT4. BD Pharmingen or ATCC for the cell lines.
6. Cell-sorting media: ice-cold Dulbecco's PBS with 2% FCS and penicillin/streptomycin. Collection tubes for sorting contain 0.5 mL FCS.
7. Plasticware. Tissue-culture flasks; 96-well U-bottom tissue culture plates; 5 mL polypropylene round-bottom tubes for cell sorting.
8. Anti-CD3 crosslinking. Use platebound anti-mouse CD3 clone 145 2C11, or platebound anti-human CD3 clone OKT3. Dilute MAb in PBS (1:1000 to 1:5,000 for purified or ascites; 1:100 for culture supernatant). Pipet 75 μL/well, then incubate 2 h at 37°C or overnight at 4°C, and wash 3× with PBS before adding cells. Prior coating of the wells with protein A, 100 μg/mL diluted in PBS, incubated 2 h at 37°C or overnight at 4°C, increases the efficiency of anti-CD3 binding.

9. Mitogens: PHA, 2 µg/mL, or conA, 4 µg/mL (Sigma). Stock solutions are prepared by dissolving PHA or conA, previously sterilized by UV or gamma irradiation, in PBS at a concentration of 1 mg/mL. Aliquots are stored frozen at –20°C.

10. Bacterial SAgs: SEA, SEB, SEC, SED, SEE, TSST-1 are used at 0.1–1 mg/mL for activation of TCRBV specific T-cell hybridomas. Stock solutions are prepared by dissolving toxins, previously sterilized by UV or gamma irradiation, in PBS at a concentration of 1 mg/mL. Aliquots are stored frozen at –20°C. SEA, SEB, and TSST-1 are available from Sigma. A complete listing of highly purified toxins is available through Toxin Technology (Sarasota, FL). **Use safety precautions when working with toxins, e.g., wear gloves and/or masks, since they are very toxic even in minute doses.**

11. Viral SAgs: APC expressing the viral SAgs are used at varying APC:responder ratios. The optimal dose is determined empirically in this way.

2.3. Cytokine ELISAs

The general protocol was adapted from BD Pharmingen.

1. Capture antibody: purified anti-cytokine MAb diluted in Binding Buffer (1–5 µg/mL). For mouse IL-2 ELISA use clone JES6-1A12 at 2 µg/mL. For human IL-2 ELISA use clone MQ1-17H12 at 2 µg/mL (BD Pharmingen).

2. Detection antibody: biotinylated anti-cytokine MAb diluted in Blocking Buffer/Tween (0.5–5 µg/mL). For mouse IL-2 ELISA use clone JES6-5H4 at 2 µg/mL. For human IL-2 ELISA use clone B33-2 at 5 µg/mL (BD Pharmingen).

3. Alkaline phosphatase conjugate: NeutrAvidin-AP (Pierce), diluted to 0.1 µg/mL in Blocking Buffer/Tween.

4. Substrate: Immunopure PNPP (*p*-nitrophenyl phosphate disodium salt) substrate solution (Pierce), made fresh each time just prior to use by adding 9.6 mL dd H_2O, 0.4 mL 5X DEA buffer (Pierce) and 1 tablet of substrate per ELISA plate.

5. Binding Buffer: 0.1 *M* Na_2HPO_4, pH 9.0.

6. Blocking Buffer/Tween: 2% BSA (immunoassay grade) in PBS, 0.4 µ filtered; then add Tween 20, 0.5 mL per liter. PBS: For 10 L, 80 g NaCl, 11.6 g Na_2HPO_4, 2 g KH_2PO_4, pH to 7.4.

7. Cytokine standards. Recombinant murine IL-2 (R&D Systems); recombinant human IL-2, (Proleukin, Chiron). Lyophilized cytokines are reconstituted according to manufacturer's suggestions in the presence of a protein carrier. Aliquots are made at concentrations of at least 10 μg/mL, and stored at –80°C. Aliquots should not be refrozen after thawing, and can be stored at 4°C for at least 1 mo. Make standard curves using twofold serial dilutions of recombinant cytokines starting from 1000 U/mL or 5000 pg/mL.

8. ELISA plates: Nunc-Immuno Plate, Maxisorp surface.

9. Equipment: ELISA plate washer (optional); ELISA plate reader for OD 405 nm; multi-pipettors.

2.4. Cytokine Bioassay

1. Cytokine dependent cell lines: HT-2 *(9)*, CTLL-2 *(12)*, Kit-225 *(13)*, are IL-2 dependent cell lines that proliferate in response to both human and mouse IL-2, (ATCC).

2. Media: RPMI supplemented with 10% FCS, glutamine, Na pyruvate, HEPES, β-Mercaptoethanol, penicillin, streptomycin (Gibco). For cell expansion, rIL-2 is added at lowest dose that enables proliferation (10–40 U/mL). Remove IL-2 from media during assay.

3. Cytokine standards. Recombinant murine IL-2 (R&D Systems); recombinant human IL-2 (Proleukin, Chiron). Lyophilized cytokines are reconstituted according to manufacturer's suggestions in the presence of a protein carrier. Aliquots are made at concentrations of at least 10 μg/mL, and stored at –80°C. Aliquots should not be refrozen after thawing, and can be stored at 4°C for at least 1 mo. Make standard curves using twofold serial dilutions of recombinant cytokines starting from 1000 U/mL or 5000 pg/mL.

4. Cell proliferation: [³H]thymidine, stock 1 mCi/mL, (NEN); dilute 1:25, then add 25 μL/well, final concentration = 1 μCi/well.

5. Harvest cells: 96-well microplates with bonded filters, e.g., UniFilter-96, GF-C (Packard). Microscint™ 20 scintillation fluid (Packard); adhesive plate sealers, or heat sealers.

6. Equipment: Tissue culture hoods and incubators (37°C, 5% CO_2); cell harvester, e.g., Packard Filtermate™; radioactivity plate scintillation counter for [³H].

3. Methods

3.1. CD69 Assay

The directions presented here assume that the investigator has significant prior experience with antibody staining and flow cytometry analysis. It is strongly recommended that the investigator test all MAbs before beginning the assay, defining the optimal staining conditions for the cells to be used prior to proceeding. It is also recommended that stimulation conditions are tested for the cells and reagents to be used prior to beginning the analysis (*see* **Note 1** and **Fig. 1**).

3.1.1. Isolation of Primary Lymphocytes

3.1.1.1. HUMAN PBMC

1. Isolate from blood using ficoll gradient density separation.
2. Wash cells twice in PBS, count and resuspend in complete RPMI media supplemented with 10% FCS at 2×10^6 cells/mL for immediate stimulation.
3. Human PBMC may be cultured overnight (*see* **Note 2**) to allow monocytes to adhere; plate at a density of 5×10^5 cells/mL in 37°C, 5% CO_2 incubator.

3.1.1.2. MOUSE LYMPHOCYTES

1. Lymph node (LN) or spleen single-cell suspensions are made by gently teasing organs in PBS or RPMI between frosted glass slides.
2. Suspension cells are then transferred to a conical tube after allowing connective tissue debris to sink due to gravity, or filtering the suspensions through Nytex to remove the debris. Spleen cells must be treated with ammonium chloride solution to thoroughly remove red blood cells, which greatly obscure FACS analysis (*see* **Note 3**).
3. Wash cells in PBS or RPMI; count and resuspend in 10% complete RPMI media at 2×10^6 cells/mL.

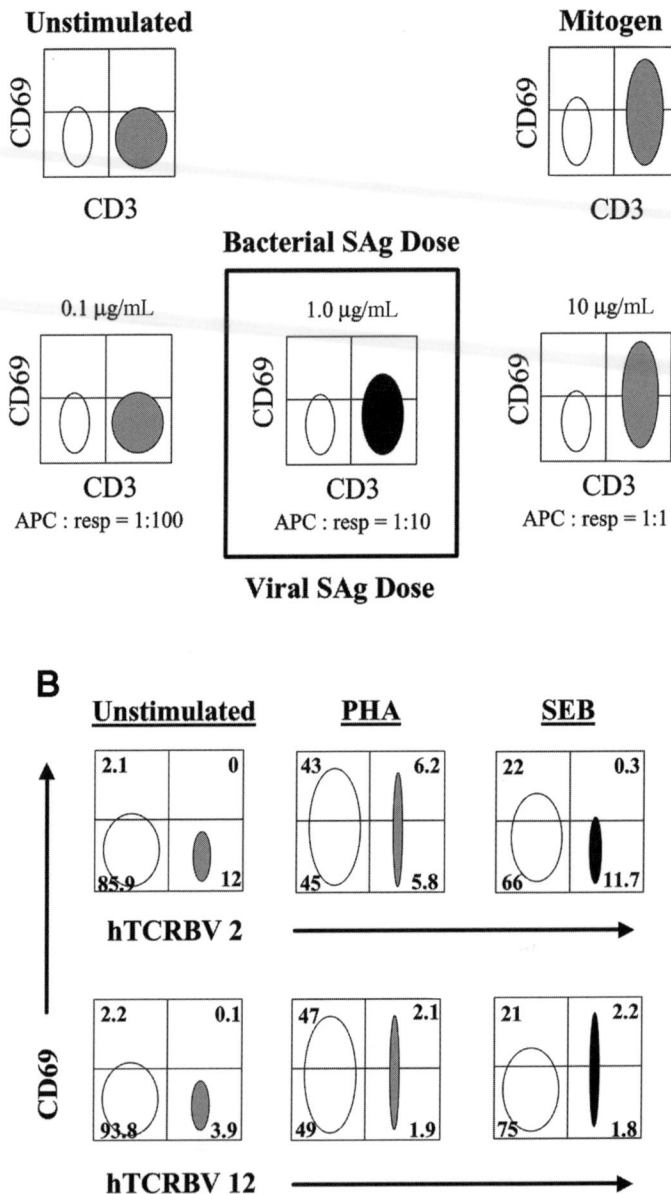

Fig.1. (**A**) Assessing proper SAg stimulation conditions for CD69 analysis. T cells are unstimulated or stimulated with mitogen, or different doses of bacterial or viral SAg. Stain cells with CD69-PE and CD3-FITC.

3.1.2. T-Cell Activation

3.1.2.1. BACTERIAL SAg STIMULATION (*SEE* FIG. 1)

1. In 6-well tissue-culture plates, add 5×10^6–10^7 lymphocytes per well
2. Adjust such that the final volume of each well is 5 mL. To one well add media only; this will be the unstimulated control. To a second well, add PHA, final concentration 2 µg/mL, for human cells; or conA, final concentration 4 µg/mL, for mouse cells; this will be the mitogenic positive control. To a third well, add bacterial SAg (*see* **Note 4** and **Fig. 1A**).
3. Cells are cultured for 3–4 h (up to 16 h, but the longer the incubation, the more background stimulation will increase) at 37°C, 5% CO_2.
4. Wash cells and resuspend in ice cold FACS buffer at a concentration of 5×10^6 cells per mL for antibody staining.

3.1.2.2. VIRAL SAg STIMULATION (*SEE* NOTE 5 AND FIG. 1)

1. Cultured APC expressing the viral SAg are washed, counted and resuspended in 10% complete RPMI media at 2×10^6 cells/mL.
2. Make 2–10-fold serial dilutions of APC expressing the viral SAg. The dose of SAg used for T-cell stimulation is varied by changing the ratio of APC:responders (*see* **Fig. 1A**). Start with an initial APC: responder ratio of 1:1 or 1:2, and serially dilute from there (*see* **Note 6**).
3. In 6-well tissue-culture plates, add 5×10^6–10^7 lymphocytes per well.
4. Add an equal number of APC to one well (APC:responder = 1:1)
5. Add serially diluted APC to additional wells (vary the APC: responder ratios).
6. Adjust such that the final volume of each well is 5 mL. For controls, to one well add media only; this will be the unstimulated control. To a second well, add PHA, final concentration 2 µg/mL, for human cells; or conA, final concentration 4 µg/mL, for mouse cells; this will be the mitogenic positive control.

Fig. 1. (*continued*) (**A**) Choose the dose of SAg that causes intermediate CD69 expression on CD3 cells. Unstimulated CD3 cells are CD69 low or negative, while approx 50% of mitogen stimulated CD3 cells are CD69 bright. (**B**) Representation of CD69 staining profile on human TCRBV2 vs TCRBV12 T-cell subsets on unstimulated cells, and 4 h PHA and SEB stimulated T cells.

3.1.3. Antibody Staining

3.1.3.1. DILUTION OF ANTIBODIES

During the incubation required for cell stimulation, calculate how many antibody stainings will be performed, and dilute the antibodies accordingly. Plan to stain unstimulated cells, mitogen stimulated cells, and SAg stimulated cells, with each anti-TCRBV MAb + anti-CD69; anti-CD3 + anti-CD69; and isotype control MAbs (these are optional, since each staining is internally controlled). The following example for a single step staining is based upon using the mouse V_β TCR Screening panel offered by BD Pharmingen. There are 17 different FITC labeled anti-TCRBV MAbs included in this panel. Optimal staining is obtained with a working dilution of 1:10 in FACS buffer, in a staining volume of 50 μL/well in a 96-well V-bottom plate. The PE labeled anti-CD69 MAb stains optimally at a working dilution of 1:50.

1. In a 5-mL tube, dilute 60 μL anti-CD69 MAb in 3 mL of FACS buffer and mix well; place on ice. This volume is sufficient for 60 stainings.
2. Label 17 (1.5 mL) Eppendorf tubes with the name of each TCRBV MAb, and label one tube with anti-CD3.
3. In each of the labeled tubes, add 160 μL of diluted anti-CD69-PE MAb; this is the volume sufficient for 3 stainings with allowance for 10% over-pipetting.
4. To each tube, add 16 μL of the individual anti-TCRBV MAb or anti-CD3 MAb. Mix well and store on ice covered from light until ready to stain.

3.1.3.2. CELL INCUBATION WITH ANTIBODY: SINGLE STEP STAINING

1. Four hour stimulated and unstimulated T cells are washed in PBS, and resuspended in FACS buffer on ice at a concentration of 5×10^6 cells/mL (*see* **Note 7**).
2. Plate 50 μL of cells/well into 96-well V-bottom plates on ice for each staining to be performed; this volume corresponds to approx 2.5×10^5 cells/well, (a range of 10^5–10^6 cells/well works fine; however, if using more than 5×10^5 cells/well, double the amount of

antibodies and staining volume to 100 µL/well). For each stimulation condition at least 20 wells are required. When using many different antibodies like this, it is easier to keep track of the staining using two 96-well plates instead of one (*see* **Fig. 2**); in addition, the second plate acts as a balance during the subsequent centrifugation steps. Pipet unstimulated cells in wells in row A of each plate; pipet mitogen stimulated cells in row B, and SAg stimulated cells in row C wells of each plate.

3. At the top of the plates above each well, label the antibody used, i.e., the particular TCRBV MAb, or anti-CD3, isotype control, and unstained control well.

4. Spin down the cells by centrifugation of the plate at 1700 rpm for 3 min at 4°C, then remove the supernatant. Resuspend the cell pellets by firmly tapping the plate, then place on ice.

5. Pipet previously diluted antibody mixtures, 50 µL/well, accordingly. After all antibodies are added, use a multi-channel pipettor to ensure that the cells and antibodies are well-mixed, changing tips between samples.

6. Incubate cells on ice covered from light for 30 min.

7. Wash cells 3 times with 200 µL of ice cold FACS buffer, with centrifugation at 1700 rpm for 3 min at 4°C.

8. Resuspend the cells in 200 µL FACS buffer then transfer cells to FACS tubes, on ice, for immediate FACS analysis; the volume in the tube can then be adjusted to whatever is optimal for the particular flow cytometry analysis instrument that is used. Alternatively, the cells can be fixed for later analysis (*see* **Subheading 3.1.3.4.**).

3.1.3.3. THREE-STEP ANTIBODY STAINING

It is possible that investigators will not have access to directly FITC-conjugated anti-TCRBV MAbs, particularly when working with the human TCR MAbs, for which a complete set does not exist. If only purified MAb are available, it is necessary to do a three-step antibody staining: first step with the purified anti-TCRBV MAb; second step with a FITC-labeled anti-mouse Ig; and third step with PE-labeled anti-CD69. If the staining is not performed sequentially, the second stage reagent will bind to both the TCRBV MAb and the anti-CD69 MAb, yielding false results (*see* **Note 8**). Staining is

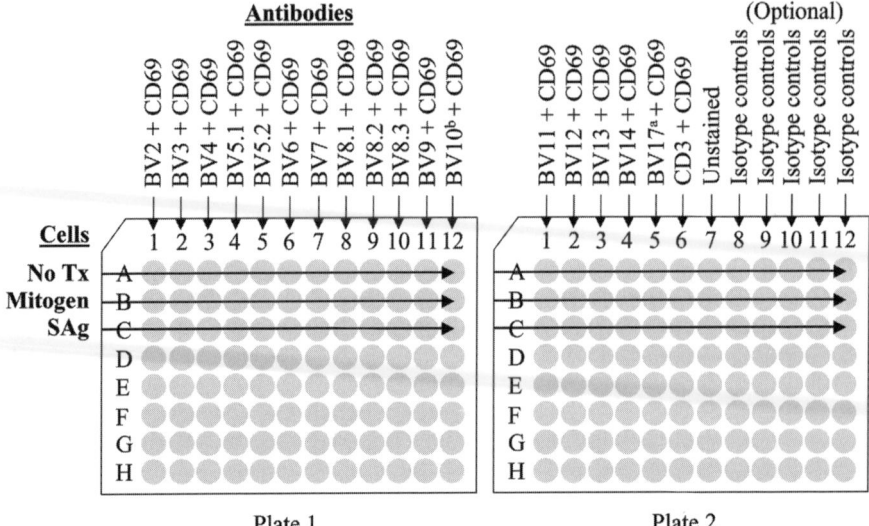

Fig. 2. Suggested scheme for antibody staining of unstimulated (No Tx), mitogen stimulated and SAg stimulated T cells for CD69 analysis of mouse TCRBV subsets. Cells are pipetted into wells of rows A–C, while antibodies are applied to wells in each numbered column, of two 96-well V-bottom plates.

performed using conditions similar to the one step staining, described in **Subheading 3.1.3.2.**, but several important issues should be considered.

1. Stain an increased number of cells/well (5×10^5–10^6), because cells are often lost during the increased number of washes that will be performed, i.e., 3 washes after the first step, 3 after the second step and 2–3 after the third step. Depending on the number of MAbs used, this may necessitate doubling the number of cells in the initial stimulation (*see* **Subheading 3.1.2.2., step 3**).
2. It is particularly important that all steps are performed on ice with sodium azide in the FACS buffer to inhibit T cell signaling by the anti-TCRBV MAbs, because of the increased length of time required for the staining procedure.
3. If using some directly conjugated anti-TCRBV MAbs and some unconjugated MAbs, add all of the primary antibodies simultaneously during the first step. During the second step, the second stage

reagent is added only to wells receiving unconjugated MAbs; FACS buffer alone is added to wells that received the FITC-conjugated primary MAbs. Anti-CD69-PE MAb is added simultaneously to all wells during the third step.

4. Because of the lengthened staining procedure, it is advisable to fix the cells, and perform the FACS analysis on a later date (*see* **Subheading 3.1.3.4.**).

3.1.3.4. CELL FIXATION

If flow cytometry cannot be performed at once, cells can be fixed without adverse consequence to the results. This is often advisable when a large experiment is performed, because the FACS analysis is time consuming. In addition, if the FACS analysis cannot be completed within several hours, cell death becomes an issue for samples that are analyzed last. Analysis can be performed on fixed cells up to a week after the staining; however, best results are obtained within 1–3 d.

1. Resuspend the cell pellets in 200 µL of 1% paraformaldehyde, diluted from a 4% stock solution in FACS buffer.
2. Incubate cells for 20 min on ice covered.
3. Wash fixed cells with FACS buffer, spin down, and resuspend in FACS buffer for postponed analysis. Store fixed cells at 4°C in the dark.

3.1.4. Flow Cytometry

1. For two-color FACS analysis, set up the following histograms: forward scatter (FSC) vs. side scatter (SSC); FSC vs FL-1 (FITC-conjugated MAb); FSC vs FL-2 (PE-conjugated MAb); and FL-1 vs FL-2.
2. Set up gates and instrument settings using the unstained controls and the anti-CD3 vs anti-CD69 controls from unstimulated and stimulated cells. In general, for unstimulated cells, less than 5% of $CD3^+$ cells express CD69 (*see* **Note 9**).
3. Draw a tight gate around the region in the FSC vs SSC histogram that contains the T-cell population, then collect at least 50,000 events within the T-cell gate for analysis (*see* **Note 10**).

4. Apply the gate to the other histograms, i.e., FSC vs FL-1, FSC vs FL-2, and FL-1 vs FL-2, because it is often difficult to identify the very small TCRBV subsets when looking at total events.

5. For each TCRBV MAb, collection should begin with the positive control, mitogen activated cells, because it is easier to compensate on the greater population of CD69^{hi} cells in each tiny TCRBV cell subset, than trying to compensate on the unstimulated cells which are CD69^{lo}, or the SAg stimulated cells which express variable levels of CD69 that differ between subsets. Analyze all cells stained with a particular anti-TCRBV MAb, before starting analysis of cells stained with other TCRBV MAbs, because compensation values often need to be adjusted for the different MAbs.

3.1.5. Analysis (See **Fig. 3**)

1. Analyze only live cells that fall within the region containing T cells on the FSC vs SSC histogram; this entails drawing a tight gate around the T-cell subset, and applying the gate to the FL-1 vs FL-2 histogram.

2. For each staining, calculate the number of CD69$^+$, TCRBV$^+$ double positive cells divided by the total number of TCRBV$^+$ cells, i.e., both CD69$^+$ and CD69$^-$ TCRBV$^+$ cells, (*see* **Note 11**).

3.2. T-Cell Hybridoma Assay

3.2.1. Maintaining T-Cell Hybridomas

Care must be taken maintaining the hybridomas to ensure that they do not spontaneously lose expression of functional TCR signaling. While the assay itself is straightforward and relatively simple, it is of crucial importance that all cell lines are growing optimally on the day of the assay, and in addition, all cell lines, media and reagents must be free of mycoplasma. Many T-cell hybridomas are inherently unstable because they are the product of a fusion of two diploid cells, resulting in an unequal duplication of chromosomes, which are frequently lost during subsequent cell divisions. The spontaneous loss of chromosomes can affect the functional ability of the cell to respond to antigen or SAg. Some hybridomas are relatively stable, yet others very rapidly lose TCR

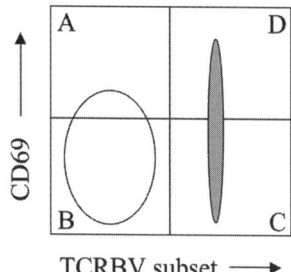

Quadrant	Gated Events	% Gated
A	12,000	20 %
B	45,000	75 %
C	1,500	2.5 %
D	1,500	2.5 %

$$\% \text{ of TCRBV subset that is } CD69^+ = D / C + D$$
$$= 1,500 / 3,000$$
$$= 50 \%$$

Fig. 3. Diagram depicting how to calculate the percentage of cells in a particular TCRBV subset that is $CD69^+$ after T-cell stimulation. 60,000 cells were collected in the lymphocyte area gate on the FSC/SSC histogram. The gated cells were analyzed for TCRBV/CD69 staining. The events collected in each quadrant (A–D) were analyzed. The percentage of cells in the TCRBV subset that stained CD69 positive are derived by dividing the number of events in quadrant D by the total number of events in quadrants C + D.

function. For this reason, it is very important that hybridomas are not maintained in vitro for any length of time other than is required to expand them for freezing early passage aliquots, or for performing the assay. It is recommended that upon obtaining a T-cell hybridoma, the investigator freeze aliquots at the *earliest* possible time point, which can be thawed out for later testing and use. If the T-cell hybridomas start to lose reactivity, it is possible to rescue the line by sorting for surface CD3 and/or CD4.

3.2.1.1. EXPAND T HYBRIDOMAS AND FREEZE ALIQUOTS

1. Upon first receiving a T-cell hybridoma, grow the cells in the recommended media, until at least 2×10^7 cells are obtained (*see* **Note 12**).
2. At the earliest possible point, freeze-down aliquots of 2×10^6 cells per freezer vial (*see* **Note 13**).

3.2.1.2. TESTING THE HYBRIDOMAS BY ANTI-CD3 CROSSLINKAGE

Each T-cell hybridoma is unique and requires particular conditions for optimal activation that can only be assessed empirically. It is necessary to test different concentrations of hybridoma cells per well and varying concentrations of APC per well. Anti-CD3 crosslinkage is considered to be a maximal stimulation for most T-cell hybridomas. Thus, optimal T hybridoma concentrations per well can be defined by varying the cell numbers on anti-CD3 coated wells, (*see* **Note 14**).

Since SAgs require MHC class II presentation, it is necessary to co-incubate hybridomas with APC and SAg; thus, the ratio of the responder (T hybridoma) to the APC needs to be determined empirically (*see* **Note 15** and **Subheading 3.2.2.**).

1. Twenty-four to forty-eight hours prior to the assay, thaw a frozen aliquot of T-cell hybridoma. If 2×10^6 cells were frozen, the thawed cells can be put into a T25 tissue-culture flask. If the assay will be performed the following day, thaw cells very early in the morning, into the appropriate media supplemented with 20% FCS. If assay will be done 2 d later, cells must be expanded the day after thawing, from the T25 flask into a T75 flask (*see* **Note 16**).
2. The day prior to the assay, coat plates with anti-CD3 MAb. Dilute antibody in PBS (for commercial preparations or ascites try dilutions of 1:1000 to 1:5000, for culture supernatant try 1:100 to 1:500), then pipet 75 µL/well into 96-well round-bottom tissue culture plates (*see* **Note 17**). A suggested scheme for testing varying concentrations of T hybridomas per well is presented in **Fig. 4**. All assay conditions should be performed using quadruplicate wells.
3. Incubate plates, wrapped in plastic to prevent evaporation, overnight at 4°C, using care to maintain sterility.
4. The day of the assay, wash anti-CD3 coated wells 3× with PBS, 200 µL/well.

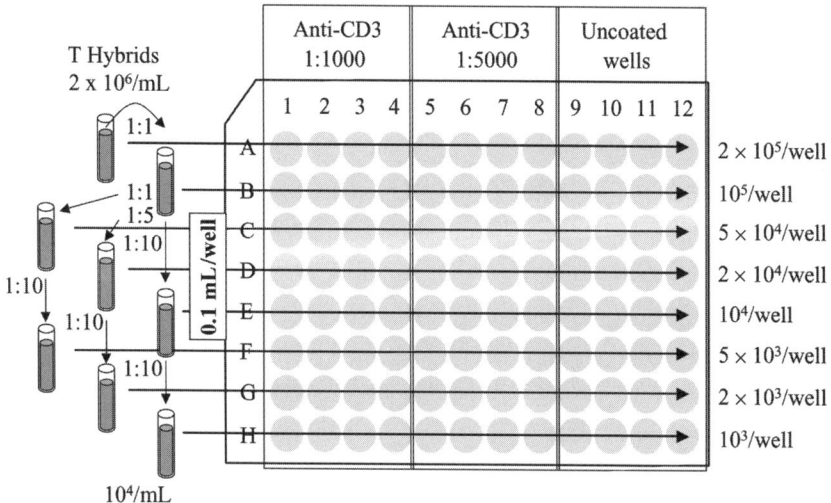

Fig. 4. Scheme for determining the optimal number of T-cell hybridomas per well for anti-CD3 cross-linkage. Start with 2×10^6 T cell hybrids/mL in a tube. Make serial dilutions as represented. Pipet the cells across rows A–H of a round bottom 96-well tissue-culture plate in which the wells were previously coated with anti-CD3 diluted 1:1,000 in PBS (columns 1–4) or 1:5,000 (columns 5–8) or were left uncoated (columns 9–12).

5. Then add media, 100 µL/well, to prevent the coated wells from drying out.
6. Count hybridoma cells and resuspend at a concentration of 2×10^6/mL.
7. Make 2 to10-fold serial dilutions ending at a concentration of 10^4/ mL.
8. Add 100 µL/well of cells from each dilution in quadruplicate wells, to anti-CD3 coated or uncoated wells. The final concentration of cells per well will thus range from a high of 2×10^5 to a low of 10^3 (*see* **Fig. 4**).
9. The final volume in each well should be 200 µL, adjust with media accordingly (*see* **Note 18**).
10. Incubate plates for 24–48 h at 37°C, 5% CO_2.
11. Freeze plates at –80°C, then test thawed supernatants for IL-2 production (*see* **Subheading 3.2.3.**).

3.2.1.3. Sorting the Hybrids for CD3 and CD4 (*see* **Fig. 5**)

If it becomes apparent that the hybridoma is losing CD3 as it is passaged, i.e., if IL-2 production significantly decreases between

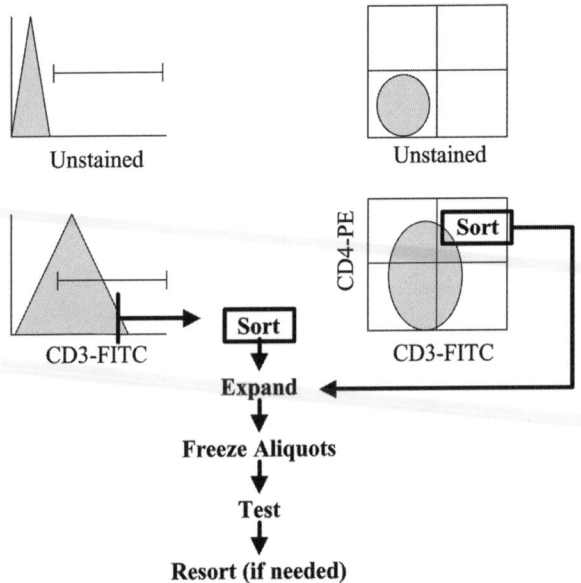

Fig. 5. Diagram depicting cell sorting of the T-cell hybrids for cells that stain CD3 bright or CD3/CD4 bright. T hybrids are stained with either CD3-FITC only, or CD3-FITC/CD4-PE. Positive cells are sorted for the top 2–3% of bright cells. These cells are expanded, then aliquots are frozen as quickly as possible. Thawed T-cell hybrids are then tested for IL-2 production after anti-CD3 cross-linkage. If IL-2 production is low, cells can be expanded and resorted.

early passage freezes and later passage freezes, it is often possible to rescue the hybridoma line by successive sorts for CD3^{hi} cells, or for CD3^{hi}/CD4^{hi} cells. Sorting should only be attempted on cells that still retain some signaling capacity, not cells that are completely nonfunctional. It is, therefore, suggested that an aliquot of *early passage* cells is used for sorting.

1. Thaw cells, and expand for several days until $2–5 \times 10^7$ cells are obtained.
2. Resuspend cells at 10^8/mL in sterile, ice cold sort buffer (PBS/2% FCS with penicillin/streptomycin).
3. Stain with FITC-labeled anti-CD3 and PE-labeled anti-CD4, diluted 1:10 in sort buffer, on ice, in the dark for 30 min.

4. Wash cells 2× with ice cold sort buffer, then resuspend in 0.5 mL of sort buffer.
5. Sort immediately, collecting the top 2–3% of cells expressing the highest levels of CD3 or CD3 + CD4 (*see* **Fig. 5**).
6. Generally, we obtain 5×10^5 cells from the sort, which are expanded for 2–3 d, yielding enough cells to make at least 10 freezer aliquots of 2×10^6 cells/vial.
7. Retest a thawed aliquot for functional TCR signaling. If IL-2 production is still low, cells can be resorted for the top 2–3%, several times successively (*see* **Note 19**).

3.2.2. SAg Stimulation of the Hybridomas

SAgs require MHC class II for presentation, and while costimulation is not necessary, it can increase T-cell activation. Probably the most difficult part of doing a T-cell hybridoma assay is coordinating the growth of the hybrids and the APC lines, such that both cell lines are growing optimally on the day of the assay. Since T-cell hybridomas cannot be maintained in vitro for long periods of time, it is useful to have a continuous supply of APC that can be readily cultured in vitro, for use when the T hybrids are ready. For this reason, many fast growing B-cell lines or MHC-transfected fibroblast lines are excellent choices for SAG presentation, particularly for the bacterial toxins that are added exogenously to co-cultures of hybrids and APC (*see* **Note 20**). However, if viral SAg will be assayed, it is necessary to use APC lines that can express the viral SAg (*see* **Note 21**).

3.2.2.1. BACTERIAL SAG STIMULATION (*SEE* FIG. 6)

It is first necessary to define the optimal APC:responder ratio. 1:1 is a good starting point for defining the optimal ratio, but it is recommended that different ratios are tested from 10:1 to 1:10, maintaining the number of hybridomas per well and the dose of toxin constant (*see* **Note 22** and **Fig. 6**). For every assay it is necessary to have a positive and negative control, and all conditions should be performed in quadruplicate. Anti-CD3 crosslinkage is a

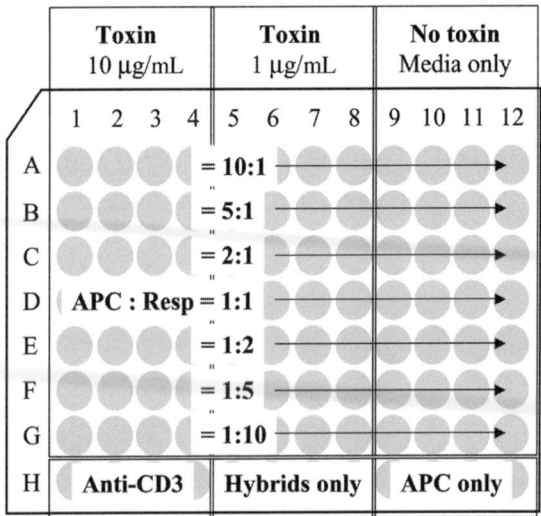

Fig. 6. Schematic for optimization of bacterial SAg stimulation of T-cell hybrids. Choose the lowest number of T hybrids per well that produced high levels of IL-2 after anti-CD3 cross-linkage. Maintain the number of T hybrids per well constant. Calculate the number of APC required for the different APC:responder ratios depicted in rows A–G. Add the required number of APC in 50 μL volume/well. Add the required number of hybrids in 50 μL volume/well. Apply 2 different doses of toxins or media only (100 μL/well) to wells in columns 1–4; 5–8; and 9–12, respectively. Pipet controls into row H: T hybrids + anti-CD3 coated wells (1–4); T hybrids + media only (5–8); APC + media only (9–12).

necessary positive control, from which can be determined the% maximal stimulation (*see* **Subheading 3.2.1.2.**). It is useful to test that the APC lines do not produce IL-2; occasionally, activated B cells secrete IL-2, which contributes to background. It is also necessary to test that the hybridomas are not stimulated by allogeneic APC in the absence of toxin.

1. Count all APC lines.
2. Decide upon the concentrations of APC used per well, and resuspend cells in media at $20 \times$ the final desired concentrations, e.g., if 2×10^4 APC/well is desired, resuspend APC at 4×10^5/mL. Refer to **Fig. 6** for a suggested scheme.
3. Make two- to fivefold serial dilutions of APC lines according to plan.

4. Pipet APC, 50 μL/ well, into 96-well round-bottom plates, using a multichannel pipetter. All conditions are performed using quadruplicate wells.

5. Count T-cell hybridomas, then resuspend in media at 20× the final concentration. e.g., if 2×10^4 hybrids/well will be used, resuspend hybrids at 4×10^5/mL.

6. Pipet 50 μL/well of the hybridomas on top of the APC.

7. Dilute the bacterial toxin in media at 2× the final concentration, e.g., if 1 μg/mL is desired, make 2 μg/mL concentration.

8. Pipet 100 μL/well of toxin, or 100 μL/well of media to negative control wells.

9. The final volume in each well should be 200 μL, adjust with media accordingly.

10. Plates are incubated for 24–48 h at 37°C, 5% CO_2.

11. Freeze plates at –80°C, then test thawed supernatants for IL-2 production (*see* **Subheading 3.2.3.**).

3.2.2.2. VIRAL SAgs STIMULATION (*SEE* FIG. 7)

Stimulation of T-cell hybrids by viral SAgs is complicated by the difficulty of not knowing how much SAg is expressed in the APC line (*see* **Note 23**). For this reason, it is necessary to test many APC:responder ratios. If doing an initial test, vary the APC:responder ratios over several logs, maintaining the number of hybrids per well constant (*see* **Fig. 7**). For every assay it is necessary to have a positive and negative control, and all conditions should be performed in quadruplicate. Anti-CD3 crosslinkage is a necessary positive control, from which can be determined the% maximal stimulation (*see* **Subheading 3.2.1.2.**). It is useful to test that the APC lines themselves do not secrete IL-2, which would contribute to background. It is also necessary to test that the hybridomas are not stimulated by allogeneic APC.

1. Count SAg-transfected APC, and untransfected or vector only transfected APC, which serve as negative controls.

2. Decide upon the concentrations of APC used per well, and resuspend cells in media at 10× the final desired concentrations, e.g., if 2×10^5 APC/well will be used, resuspend APC at 2×10^6/mL. Refer to **Fig. 7** for a suggested scheme.

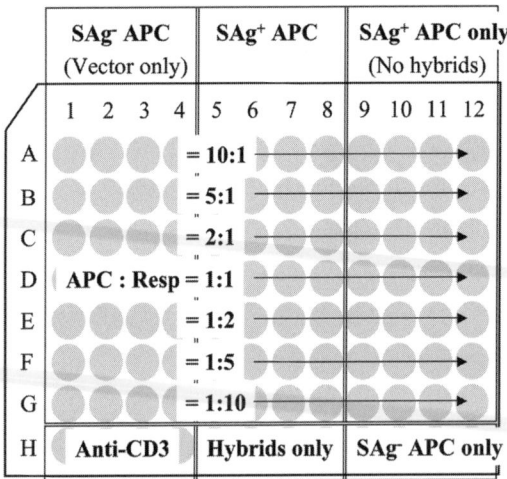

	SAg⁻ APC (Vector only)	SAg⁺ APC	SAg⁺ APC only (No hybrids)

Fig. 7. Schematic for optimization of viral SAg stimulation of T cell hybrids. Choose the lowest number of T hybrids per well that produced high levels of IL-2 after anti-CD3 cross-linkage. Maintain the number of T hybrids per well constant. (A second plate can be done simultaneously using 5× the number of T hybrids in plate 1.) Calculate the number of APC expressing viral SAg (SAg⁺ APC) or SAg negative APC (untransfected cells or APC transfected with vector only) that are required for the different APC : responder ratios depicted in rows A–G. Add the required number of APC in 100 µL volume/well (SAg⁻, columns 1–4, or SAg⁺, columns 5–12). Add the required number of hybrids in 100 µL volume/well (columns 1–8), or media only 100 µL/well (columns 9–12). Pipet controls into row H: T hybrids + anti-CD3 coated wells (1–4); T hybrids + media only (5–8); SAg⁻ APC + media only (9–12).

3. Make serial dilutions of APC lines according to plan.
4. Pipet APC, 100 µL/ well, into 96-well round-bottom plates.
5. Count T-hybridoma cell lines.
6. Resuspend hybrids in media at 10× the final concentration, e.g., if 2×10^4 hybrids/well will be used, resuspend hybrids at 2×10^5/mL.
7. Pipet 100 µL/well of the hybridomas on top of the APC.
8. The final volume in each well should be 200 µL, adjust accordingly.
9. Plates are incubated for 24–48 h at 37°C, 5% CO_2.
10. Freeze plates at –80°C, then test thawed supernatants for IL-2 production (see **Subheading 3.2.3.**).

3.2.3. Cytokine Assays

3.2.3.1. ELISA

Cytokine detection ELISAs are the most consistent means for measuring IL-2 production. Thaw frozen hybridoma cell supernatants at room temperature (RT) or 37°C. Freezing disrupts the cell pellet, releasing intracellular IL-2 into the media. One half of the supernatant (100 μL/well) should be tested. Refreeze the leftover supernatants, which can be retested if problems arise. The results must be compared with a standard curve using serial twofold dilutions of recombinant IL-2 in the range of 1000 U/mL (5000 pg/mL), to 0.1 U/mL (0.5 pg/mL).

1. Dilute capture antibody to 2 μg/mL in binding solution.
2. Coat ELISA plates with 50 μL/well.
3. Seal and incubate plates overnight at 4°C.
4. Wash 4× with PBS/Tween, 200 μL/well.
5. Add Blocking Buffer, 200 μL/well.
6. Seal and incubate 30 min RT (or 4°C overnight).
7. Wash 3× with PBS/Tween.
8. Dilute standards in Blocking Buffer/Tween.
9. Add thawed supernatant samples and standards, 100 μL/well.
10. Seal and incubate 2 h at RT.
11. Wash plate 4× with PBS/Tween.
12. Dilute detection antibody to 2 μg/mL in Blocking Buffer/Tween.
13. Add 100 μL/well.
14. Seal and incubate 1 h at RT.
15. Wash 6× with PBS/Tween.
16. Dilute Neutravidin-AP to 0.1 mg/mL in Blocking Buffer/Tween.
17. Add 100 μL/well.
18. Seal and incubate at RT for 30 min.
19. Wash 8× with PBS/Tween.
20. Prepare substrate solution immediately prior to use, add 100 μL/well.
21. Incubate at RT in the dark, watching periodically for color development (15–30 min).
22. Read OD at 405 nm.

3.2.3.2. BIOASSAY

IL-2 in the cell supernatants can be measured by testing for proliferation of an IL-2 dependent cell line, such as HT-2. Thaw frozen hybridoma cell supernatants at RT or 37°C. Freezing disrupts the cell pellet, releasing intracellular IL-2 into the media. One half of the supernatant (100 µL/well) should be tested, refreezing the leftover, which can be retested if problems arise. The results must be compared with a standard curve using serial twofold dilutions of recombinant IL-2 in the range of 1000 U/mL (5000 pg/mL), to 0.1 U/mL (0.5 pg/mL).

1. Twenty-four to forty-eight hours prior to the assay, expand HT-2 cells in 10% complete RPMI media, supplemented with recombinant IL-2 (10–40 U/mL) (*see* **Note 24**).
2. On the day of the assay, wash HT-2 cells with PBS to remove IL-2.
3. Count cells, and resuspend in media *lacking IL-2* at a concentration of 2×10^5 cells/mL.
4. Pipet HT-2 cells, 100 µL/well, into 96-well round-bottom tissue culture plates (final concentration is 2×10^4 cells/well).
5. Pipet thawed supernatant samples, 100 µL/well, on top of HT-2 cells.
6. Serially dilute recombinant IL-2 in media, to construct a standard curve.
7. Pipet 100 µL/well onto HT-2 cells, in quadruplicate wells.
8. The final volume in all wells should be 200 µL, adjust accordingly.
9. Incubate cells overnight at 37°C, 5% CO_2.
10. The next morning, pulse cells with [^{3}H]thymidine, 1 µCi/well.
11. Incubate 6 h at 37°C.
12. Harvest cells, and count for [^{3}H]thymidine incorporation.

4. Notes

1. This can be accomplished by staining with anti-CD3 MAb in place of the panel of TCRBV MAbs, greatly reducing FACS time, and conserving expensive MAbs. If the stimulation is too high, the entire CD3$^+$ T-cell population will express CD69, and therefore differences between individual TCRBV subsets cannot be identified, e.g., this occurs after 1 h stimulation with the phorbol ester PMA, where 100% of CD3$^+$ cells express CD69. Mitogen

stimulation with PHA or conA is an ideal positive control, resulting in CD69 expression on approx 50% of CD3$^+$ lymphocytes after
3–4 h, while expression is typically well below 5% for unstimulated
cells (*see* **Fig. 1A**). The conditions for SAg stimulation need to be
adjusted so that CD69 levels are not so high that differences
between the TCRBV subsets will be missed. On the other hand, if
the SAg stimulation is not high enough, the CD69 profile will
resemble that of unstimulated cells with very few of the T cells
expressing CD69. Best results will be obtained when approx 10–30%
of CD3$^+$ T cells express CD69, after stimulation with a particular
dose of SAg (*see* **Fig 1A**). Once the ideal conditions for SAg stimulation are determined with anti-CD3 staining, the assay is begun
using the entire panel of TCRBV MAbs (*see* **Fig 1B**).

2. Overnight culture is optional; we find it results in reduced background T-cell activation, and may thus be preferable for certain
applications.

3. It may be preferable to enrich for T lymphocytes in spleen cell preparations, but not absolutely necessary. Because additional steps are
required for assessing splenic T-cell activation, it is strongly recommended that LN cells are used when first attempting CD69 assays.

4. It is highly recommended that the assay is initially performed using
a well-characterized bacterial toxin, such as SEB, added at a final
concentration of 1 μg/mL, if partially purified, as is that obtained
from Sigma, (highly purified toxins can be added at 10–100-fold
lower concentrations). For bacterial toxins, there are sufficient
endogenous APC present in PBMC or LN preparations for efficient
SAg presentation.

5. It is not recommended that investigators begin testing viral SAgs,
until they have obtained consistent results with a well-characterized
bacterial SAg. For each assay it is necessary to include unstimulated
control cells, and mitogen stimulated control cells.

6. It is possible to identify the ideal ratio initially by staining with anti-
CD3 in place of the panel of TCRBV MAbs, thus reducing FACS
time, and conserving expensive MAbs. If the APC:responder ratio is
too high, the entire CD3$^+$ T cell population will express CD69, and
therefore differences between individual subsets cannot be identified.
On the other hand, if the APC:responder ratio is too low, the CD69
profile will resemble that of unstimulated cells with very few of the
T cells expressing CD69. Best results will be obtained when approx
10–30% of CD3$^+$ T cells express CD69, after stimulation with a

particular dose of viral SAg. Once the ideal dose of viral SAg is determined, the assay is repeated using the entire panel of TCRBV MAbs.

7. It is crucial that all steps are performed on ice, in the presence of
sodium azide, which prevents capping and internalization, in order
to inhibit T-cell signaling. The anti-TCRBV MAbs under certain
conditions can stimulate the T cells to express CD69, thus obscuring
the results.

8. Because the anti-TCRBV MAbs bind very small subsets of T cells,
on average 0.5–5%, it is very important that the second stage reagent
is optimally diluted. We have found that Zymed second stage
reagents at working dilutions of 1:1000 or 1:2000 give optimal staining with low background, despite the manufacturer's suggestion of
using dilutions of 1:10 or 1:20. At these higher concentrations, the
background staining often usurps the specific staining of the very
small T-cell subsets. Therefore, it is advised that prior to beginning a
CD69 assay, the investigator should first test out the different anti-
TCRBV MAbs with the second stage reagents using T-cell samples
that are not crucially important or difficult to obtain, to ensure that
consistent staining profiles are detected.

9. On mitogen activated cells, approx half of CD3$^+$ cells express CD69
after 3–4 h; however, as stated earlier, the CD69 profile on CD3$^+$
cells after SAg stimulation varies greatly, depending on the dose of
SAg and the individual SAg used. If CD69 expression is either too
high or too low on SAG stimulated CD3$^+$ cells, it may not be worth
continuing the analysis. If SAG stimulation was too strong or pro-
gressed for too long a time, the entire CD3$^+$ T-cell population will
express CD69, and therefore differences between individual TCRBV
subsets cannot be identified. On the other hand, if the SAg stimulation was too weak, the CD69 profile will resemble that of
unstimulated cells with very few of the T cells expressing CD69.
Best results will be obtained when approx 10–30% of CD3$^+$ T cells
express CD69 after SAg stimulation. If the CD69 profile of CD3$^+$
cells falls within this approximate range, continue with the analysis
of the TCRBV MAbs.

10. Because the individual TCRBV subsets comprise a very small percentage of the total lymphocytes, generally 0.5–3% for humans, and
0.5–10% for mice, it is crucial that many more events are collected
than would be for a traditional analysis. Thus, very large files are
created if all events are saved, particularly when contaminating red

cells or many dead cells are present, which are also counted as events. This can result in problems during the analysis if too many events are collected, because many analysis programs are unable to analyze more than 200,000 events; therefore, in these cases, only the events falling within the T-cell gate should be saved.

11. Assuming that the FITC-anti-TCRBV MAb is shown on the x axis, and the PE-anti-CD69 MAb is shown on the y axis, this is obtained by dividing the number of events collected in the top right quadrant, by the total number of gated events collected in the top and bottom right quadrants (*see* **Fig. 3**). For unstimulated cells, the ratios should be extemely low for each of the TCRBV MAbs used. For the positive control, mitogen-stimulated cells, the ratios should be much higher, approx 50%, and uniformly similar for each TCRBV MAb used. On the other hand, significant differences should be obtained in the ratios for SAg stimulated cells. Preferential expression of CD69 on particular TCRBV subsets is characteristic of SAg stimulation.

12. Do not allow hybridomas to overgrow prior to freezing. Healthy cells divide very rapidly, and frequently expand 10-fold overnight. Most hybridomas are contact-sensitive, thus it is recommended that cell density not exceed $2–3 \times 10^5$ cells/mL. Cells that are not growing optimally will die during the freezing process.

13. It is not recommended that cells are maintained in vitro for longer than 1 wk of culture, and the least amount of time spent in culture is best. Aliquots of 2×10^6 cells per vial on average allows investigators to thaw the cells 1–2 d prior to performing the assay, yielding a suitable number of cells with which to perform the assay. It is suggested that as many early passage aliquots as possible are frozen immediately. An aliquot of frozen cells should be thawed and tested for the conditions that produce optimal IL-2 production with controlled stimuli, prior to testing unknown samples for stimulation. Once optimal stimulation conditions are known, it can be assumed that all aliquots frozen simultaneously will yield reproducible results if assays are performed in the same manner.

14. In general, 2×10^4 T hybridomas per well yields good IL-2 production, but one should test within the range of one log higher and lower for optimal results. Choose the lowest concentration of cells per well that gives high activation, because in subsequent experiments APC will be added to the wells resulting in competition for media growth factors.

15. Assaying viral SAg requires testing APC that express the viral SAg. Since the dose of viral SAg is always unknown, many different APC:responder ratios must be tested. It is much easier to assess activation by bacterial SAgs, since the toxins can be added at known concentrations to the wells.

16. Healthy hybridomas usually expand up to 10-fold overnight, and it is important that the cells are not allowed to overgrow because they rapidly apoptose. On the day of the assay, the hybridomas should be growing optimally (cell density less than $2-3 \times 10^5$/cells/mL media). Trypan blue staining should yield fewer than 1% blue cells.

17. If antibody is limiting, e.g., if using culture supernatant, it may be necessary to first coat the plates with protein A to enhance antibody binding. Dilute protein A in PBS to a final concentration of 100 µg/mL, then pipet 75 µL/well. Incubate plates at 37°C for 2 h, then wash plates 3 times with PBS, 200 µL/well, before adding the diluted anti-CD3 MAb. Incubate overnight at 4°C.

18. Leftover hybridoma cells may be immediately frozen or expanded for use the following day, but should not be maintained in vitro for any length of time, because they so rapidly lose functional TCR signaling capacity. It is crucially important to keep track of the amount of time the hybridomas have been maintained in vitro. If the cells are refrozen, the passage number should be indicated on the freezer vial. It cannot be assumed that freezes from different passages will behave in a functionally similar manner. Instead, an aliquot from each passage needs to be retested for functional TCR signaling.

19. Each sort should increase the level of CD3 on the surface of the cell, which can be seen on the FL1 vs FL2 histogram. Since it is a log scale, small increases in fluorescence, can actually depict large differences in functionality. However, it should be cautioned that sorting does not always restore functional signaling, even if the level of CD3 obviously increases. This is likely due to other downstream signaling defects that can occur in the inherently unstable hybridomas. If repeated sorting does not restore function, toss out the cells and sort another early passage freezer aliquot.

20. Although SAgs are dependent on MHC class II, they are not restricted to a particular haplotype, and can be presented to T-cell hybridomas by xenogeneic class II molecules. Both mouse and human B-cell lines make good APC, and there are a number of fibro-

blast lines transfected with mouse or human MHC class II genes that are also useful.

21. Since the best characterized viral SAg, Mls-1, is toxic and is expressed at very low levels in the cell, APC cannot be stained with MAbs specific for Mls. Instead, it is necessary to look for transcription of the gene in stable transfectants. Because the transfectants can spontaneously stop expressing the SAg during in vitro culture, it is important to make early passage freezer aliquots of the SAg transfected APC lines, as were made for the T-cell hybridomas.

22. For an initial test, one should vary the APC number maintaining the dose of toxin stable, e.g., at 1 μg/mL, a generally high enough dose of most toxins to activate most hybrids. In general for bacterial toxin presentation, defining the optimal APC:responder ratio is less important than for viral SAg presentation, and many ratios will be capable of presenting high dose toxin. Presentation of low-dose toxin is more dependent upon the identification of optimal conditions for presentation, and for this costimulation may become an issue. Addition of activating anti-CD28 antibodies to the hybridomas can sometimes increase production of cytokine.

23. The best indication for SAg expression is transcription, since MAbs are not sensitive enough for SAg detection. Northern blotting of transfected cell lines for SAg transcripts is recommended. Bicistronic expression vectors containing marker genes, such as *EGFP* (enhanced green fluorescent protein) in the second cistron, and the SAg in the first cistron, are also useful for indicating SAg transcription. EGFP[+] cells that express the SAg transcripts can be isolated by cell sorting. Making EGFP fusion proteins or applying his tags, etc., to the N- or C-termini of the *SAg* gene is *not recommended*. In our hands, attempts at modifying the ends of Mls protein has abrogated the ability of the SAg to functionally activate T cells. Alternatively, APC can sometimes be induced to express endogenous SAg. IL-4 treatment of mouse B cell lines has been shown to upregulate Mls *(14)*, and phorbol ester and IFN-α treatment enhances presentation of the EBV associated SAg, HERV-K18 Env *(3,15,16)* in infected human B-cell lines.

24. HT-2 cells grow very rapidly; they are contact sensitive and must be split 1:100 every 2 d, requiring the addition of fresh IL-2 to the media.

References

1. Herman, A., Kappler, J. W., Marrack, P., and Pullen, A. M. (1991) Superantigens: mechanism of T-cell stimulation and role in immune responses. *Annu. Rev. Immunol.* **9,** 745–772.
2. Testi, R., Pulcinelli, F., Frati, L., Gazzaniga, P. P., and Santoni, A. (1990) CD69 is expressed on platelets and mediates platelet activation and aggregation. *J. Exp. Med.* **172,**701–707.
3. Sutkowski, N., Palkama, T., Ciurli, C., Sekaly, R. P., Thorley-Lawson, D. A., and Huber, B. T. (1996) An Epstein-Barr virus-associated superantigen. *J. Exp. Med.* **184,** 971–980.
4. Waller, E. K., Sen-Majumdar, A., Kamel, O. W., Hansteen, G. A., Schick, M. R., and Weissman, I. L. (1992) Human T-cell development in SCID-hu mice: staphylococcal enterotoxins induce specific clonal deletions, proliferation, and anergy. *Blood* **80,** 3144–3156.
5. Baribaud, F., Wirth, S., Maillard, I., Valsesia, S., Acha-Orbea, H., and Diggelmann, H. (2001) Identification of key amino acids of the mouse mammary tumor virus superantigen involved in the specific interaction with T-cell receptor V(beta) domains. *J. Virol.* **75,** 7453–7461.
6. Melchers, F., Potter, M., and Warner, N. L. (1978) Lymphocyte hybridomas. Second workshop on "functional properties of tumors of T and B lymphocytes." Preface. *Curr. Top. Microbiol. Immunol.* **81,** IX–XXIII.
7. Kouttab, N., Tannir, N., Pathak, S., Berger, A., Sahasrabuddhe, C. G., and Maizel, A. L. (1985) Establishment of stable human T-T hybridomas. *J. Immunol. Methods* **77,** 165–172.
8. Choi, Y. W., Herman, A., DiGiusto, D., Wade, T., Marrack, P., and Kappler, J. (1990) Residues of the variable region of the T-cell-receptor beta-chain that interact with S. aureus toxin superantigens. *Nature* **346,** 471–473.
9. Kappler, J. W., Skidmore, B., White, J., and Marrack, P. (1981) Antigen-inducible, H-2-restricted, interleukin-2-producing T cell hybridomas. Lack of independent antigen and H-2 recognition. *J. Exp. Med.* **153,** 1198–1214.
10. Norcross, M. A., Bentley, D. M., Margulies, D. H., and Germain, R. N. (1984) Membrane Ia expression and antigen-presenting accessory cell function of L cells transfected with class II major histocompatibility complex genes. *J. Exp. Med.* **160,** 1316–1337.

11. Mix, D. and Winslow, G. (1996) Proteolytic processing activates a viral superantigen. *J. Exp. Med.* **184,** 1549–1554.
12. Conlon, P. J. (1983) A rapid biologic assay for the detection of interleukin 1. *J. Immunol.* **131,** 1280–1282.
13. Hori, T., Uchiyama, T., Tsudo, M., Umadome, H., Ohno, H., Fukuhara, S., et al. (1987) Establishment of an interleukin 2-dependent human T cell line from a patient with T cell chronic lymphocytic leukemia who is not infected with human T cell leukemia/lymphoma virus. *Blood* **70,** 1069–1072.
14. Beutner, U., Rudy, C., and Huber. B. T. (1992) Molecular characterization of Mls-1. *Int. Rev. Immunol.* **8,** 279–288.
15. Sutkowski, N., Conrad, B., Thorley-Lawson, D. A., and Huber, B. T. (2001) Epstein-Barr virus transactivates the human edogenous retrovirus HERV-K18 that encodes a superantigen. *Immunity* **15,** 579–589.
16. Staufer, Y., Marguerat, S., Meylan, F., Ucla, C., Sutkowski, N., Huber, B. T., Pelet, T., and Conrad, B. (2001) Interferon-α induced endogenous superantigen: a model link between the environment and autoimmunity. *Immunity* **15,** 591–601.

14

Superantigen-Induced Changes in Epithelial Ion Transport and Barrier Function

Use of an In Vitro Model

James L. Watson and Derek M. McKay

1. Introduction

The small intestine selectively absorbs digested macromolecules, vitamins, minerals, and electrolytes, whereas the large intestine supports the majority of the gut microflora and reabsorbs water. These activities are the primary functions of the intestinal epithelium, a single layer of cells (principally transporting enterocytes, but also goblet cells, Paneth cells, enteroendocrine cells, and microfold "M" cells) that line the gut and interface directly with the contents of the lumen —effectively, the external environment. As such, the intestinal epithelium comprises a physical barrier that, in concert with nutrient absorption, must manage the transport of antigenic stimuli and prevent the incursion of potentially pathogenic organisms. The gut is continuously exposed to a high load of potentially noxious material derived from the diet and gut microflora, so it is not surprising that the intestine contains a large proportion of the body's immune cells and is effectively the body's largest immune organ.

From: *Methods in Molecular Biology, vol. 214: Superantigen Protocols*
Edited by: T. Krakauer © Humana Press Inc., Totowa, NJ

Although homoeostatic control of epithelial function has historically been considered the responsibility of the neuro-endocrine system, it is now evident that immune cells and their products (e.g., cytokines) influence many aspects of epithelial activity including: permeability (e.g., barrier), ion transport, and mediator release *(1–4)*. Also, bacteria and their products are known to directly affect epithelial physiology *(5)*. Moreover, a wealth of data has been amassed implicating the commensal microflora in intestinal inflammatory disorders, including Crohn's disease *(6)*.

Superantigens (SAg) are microbe-produced, low molecular-weight proteins capable of initiating T-cell activation *en masse*. T-cell activation by conventional antigen is governed by T-cell receptor (TCR) "recognition" of antigen complexed with major histocompatibility class (MHC) molecules; most antigens are recognized by only a small fraction (0.002%) of the total-body T-cell population. SAg override this interaction by binding beyond the antigen-specific groove to the variable portion of the β-chain of the TCR and similarly on an outside domain of the MHCII subunit, causing polyclonal T-cell activation that can directly activate up to 25% of all T cells. Toxic shock syndrome (TSS) is caused by the *Staphylococcus aureus*-produced SAg TSST-1, and there is evidence that bacterial SAg are involved in multisystem vasculitis (Kawasaki syndrome) *(7)*. Moreover, SAg may be involved in a number of inflammatory disorders including insulin-dependent diabetes mellitus, arthritis, celiac disease, and Crohn's disease *(7)*. We have shown, in cell culture and in rodents, that the superantigens *S. aureus* enterotoxin B (SEB) and *Yersinia pseudotuberculosis* mitogen (YPM) have the ability to perturb epithelial cell function by reducing ion-secretion events, increasing epithelial permeability, and altering jejunal architecture *(8–11)*. However, mechanistic definition of SAg action on epithelial physiology by experimentation in vivo or with explanted tissue segments is confounded by the inherent complexity of the gut mucosa. The use of in vitro culture models offers the opportunity to study cell-cell or cell-mediator interactions (that may go unnoticed in vivo) in a controlled, defined environment *(12,13)*. Though not without caveats, cultured cell lines and the use of isolated cells have the advantages of being homotypic, readily available, and often well-characterized, and in vitro models allow the investigator precise control over experimental and environmental variables *(14)*. Here we outline an approach to examine the nature of SAg-immune cell interactions on cultured intestinal epithelial cells.

2. Materials

2.1. Solutions

1. 10X Phosphate-buffered saline (PBS): 80.0 g NaCl, 2.0 g KCl, 2.0 g KH$_2$PO$_4$, 11.5 g Na$_2$HPO$_4$·7H$_2$O or 4.9 g Na$_2$HPO$_4$, 0.5 g NaN$_3$. Add dH$_2$O to 1 L, autoclave (121°C, 15 min) or filter to sterilize. Store at 4°C or room temperature. Dilute 50 mL in 450 mL sterile dH$_2$O for 1X solution.

2. Kreb's buffer: 6.72 g NaCl, 0.60 g KCl, 0.14 g CaCl$_2$, 0.11 g MgCl$_2$, 0.27 g KH$_2$PO$_4$, 2.1 g NaHCO$_3$, 1.8 g D-glucose. Add dH$_2$O to 1 L, store at 4°C. *Immediately prior to use, first oxygenate (10 min) then pH to 7.33–7.37 using 1 N HCl and 1 N NaOH. Note: To minimize the risk of contamination, omit glucose and add (10 mM) prior to use.

3. T84 medium: 1:1 (v/v) Dulbeco's modified Eagle's medium (DMEM)/Ham's F12 medium supplemented with 2% (v/v) NaHCO$_3$, 200 mM L-glutamine, 2% (v/v) penicillin-streptomycin, 1.5% (w/v) HEPES, 10% (v/v) fetal calf serum (FCS) as culture medium. Keep sterile and store at 4°C, viable ~3 mo.

4. 10X Hank's balanced salt solution (HBSS): 80.0 g NaCl, 4.0 g KCl, 0.9 g Na$_2$HPO$_4$·7H$_2$O, 0.6 g KH$_2$PO$_4$, 3.5 g NaHCO$_3$, 1.4 g CaCl$_2$, 1.0 g MgCl$_2$·6H$_2$O, 1.0 g MgSO$_4$·7H$_2$O, 10.0 g D-glucose. Add dH$_2$O to 1 L, autoclave (121°C, 15 min) or filter to sterilize. Store at 4°C. Note: All buffers and media are available from Sigma (St. Louis, MO) or Gibco-BRL/Life Technologies Inc. (Rockville, MD).

2.2. Cell Types

1. Epithelial cells: A number of human (T84, HT-29, CaCo-2, SW460) and rodent (MODE K, IEC-6, IEC-18, KATO III) immortalized,

transformed, or tumor cell lines are commercially available (American type culture collection [ATCC]; Manassas, VA), the individual phenotypes of which facilitate the investigation of different phenomena (*see* **Note 1**). Another consideration is the use of enterocytes freshly isolated from animal or human resected tissue. Historically, primary cells have been suitable for use only in short-term experiments (i.e., hours), but improvements in culture techniques now allow for longer-term culture *(15)*. For isolation and culture methodology for gut epithelia, *see* Pang et al. *(16)*.

2. Immune cells: We have primarily used peripheral blood mononuclear cells (PBMC) from human volunteers (*see* **Note 2**). Depending on the application, it may be more appropriate to select gut-derived immune cells (i.e., lamina propria mononuclear cells [LPMC]), since these cells are known to differ from PBMC in a number of properties *(17)*. An additional option is the use of established hematopoetic cell lines, such as Jurkat T cells or THP-1 monocytes.

2.3. Cell Culture

1. Cell-culture medium: DMEM, minimal essential medium (MEM), Ham's F12; supplements: fetal calf serum (FCS), antibiotics (penicillin-streptomycin), sodium bicarbonate, sodium pyruvate, HEPES, L-glutamine (*see* **Note 3**), 0.25% Trypsin-EDTA.
2. Plastic-ware, including sterile 75 cm^2 tissue-culture flasks, 60, 100, or 150 mm diameter plates, 6-, 12-, and 24-well plates.
3. Transwell plates (Costar Inc., Cambridge, MA) (*see* **Note 4**). Note: It is critical that all nonsterile materials (e.g. Pasteur pipets) be autoclaved (121°C, 15 min).

2.4. Immune Cell Isolation and Activation

1. Hepranized blood collection tubes.
2. Ficoll-Paque PLUS (PBMC isolation) and iso-osmotic Percoll (LPMC isolation) (both from Amersham Pharmacia Biotech, Piscataway, NJ).
3. Wire-mesh screens, plastic-ware.
4. 10-mL syringes and needles.
5. Bacterial products (e.g., SEB) and cell mitogens (12-phorbol-13-myristic acid [PMA]).

2.5. Major Apparatus

1. Cell-culture apparatus: desktop centrifuge (swing bucket, accepts 15- and 50-mL tubes), laminar flow hood with aspirator, heated CO_2 incubator, heated water bath, standard or inverted microscope.
2. Voltmeter with chopstick electrodes (Millicell-ERS, Millipore, Bedford, MA) to monitor transepithelial resistance (TER).
3. Ussing chambers (World Precision Instruments (WPI), Sarasota, FL) and Voltage Clamp (DVC-100; WPI), including tubing and agar bridges, matched pre-amplifiers and calomel electrodes, heating pump, aeration regulator, chart recorder, or computerized acquisition system.

3. Methods

3.1. Cell Culture

We grow and passage T84 human colon-carcinoma cells in 75 cm^2 tissue-culture flasks under standard growth conditions (37°C, 5% CO_2) using T84 media (*see* **Subheading 2.3., step 1**) replaced twice weekly.

1. Cells are passaged (*see* **Note 5**) at confluence (*see* **Note 6**) (usually 7–10 d after seeding), returning approx 1.5×10^7 cells to a new flask.
2. Cells are counted using a standard haemocytometer slide and microscope (*see* **Note 7**).

When seeding onto transwell filter supports, we typically seed at 10^6 cells/filter, where the filter size is 1 cm^2 (12-well plate) (*see* **Note 8**) in 1 mL media, with 1.5–2.0 mL media added to the basal chamber (*see* **Fig. 1**). While being cultured on transwells, media should be changed the day after seeding and every 24–48 h thereafter. By this method, T84 cells generally take 5–10 d to set up a maximally tight electrical resistance (1000–3000 Ω/cm^2) (*see* **Note 9**).

3.2. Immune Cell Isolation

3.2.1. PBMC Isolation

We have used both peripheral blood mononuclear cells (PBMC) and lamina propria (LPMC) cells for activation by SAg. The fol-

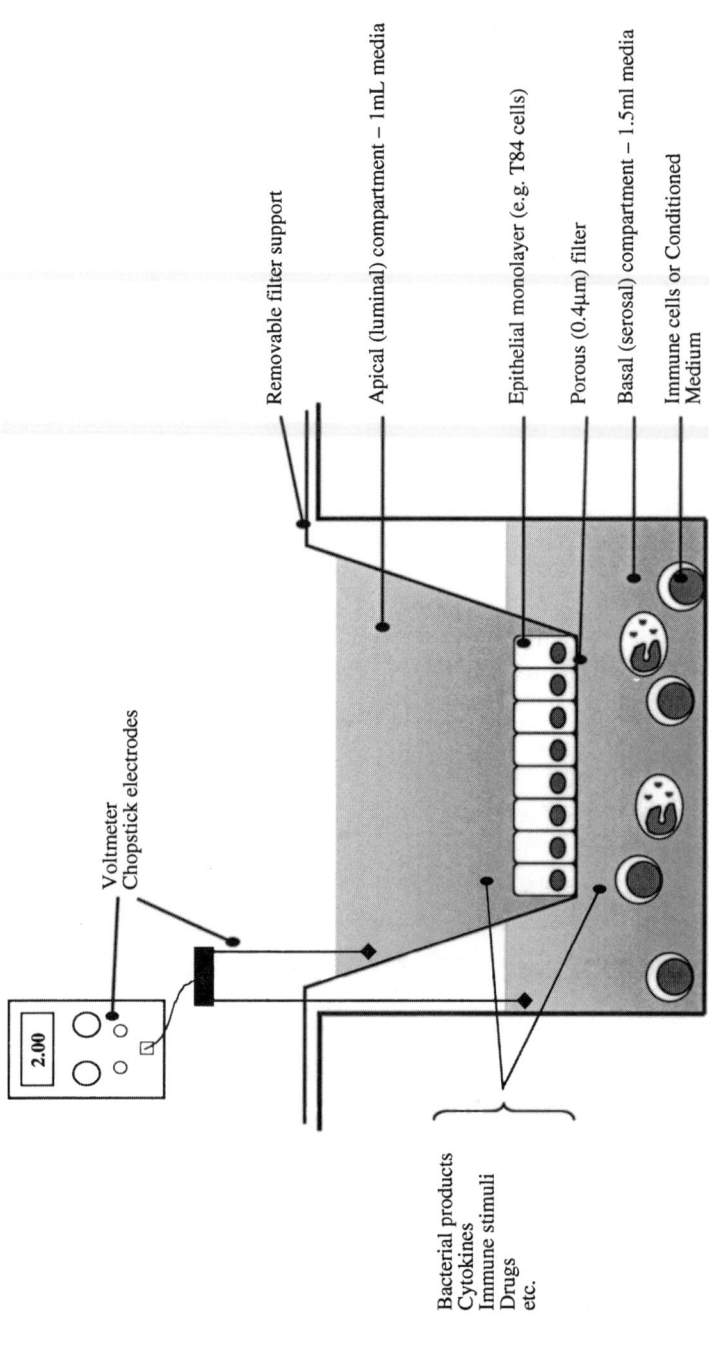

Removable filter support

Apical (luminal) compartment – 1mL media

Epithelial monolayer (e.g. T84 cells)

Porous (0.4μm) filter

Basal (serosal) compartment – 1.5ml media

Immune cells or Conditioned Medium

Voltmeter
Chopstick electrodes

2.00

Bacterial products
Cytokines
Immune stimuli
Drugs
etc.

Fig. 1. Standard transwell in vitro set-up showing epithelial cells cultured on filter support with distinct apical and basal compartments (not to scale).

lowing describes an inexpensive technique to isolate PBMC from donor blood using a Ficoll-Paque density gradient.

1. ~10 mL of venus blood is collected in heparinized tubes.
2. The following steps must be conducted under sterile conditions.
3. Transfer blood to a 50-mL plastic tube containing 10 mL pre-warmed (37°C) sterile PBS.
4. An underlay is prepared using a Pasteur pipet to slowly deliver 10 mL Ficoll (*see* **Note 10**) solution to the bottom of the tube (*see* **Fig. 2**).
5. Being careful not to disturb the layering, tubes are centrifuged for 40 min at 300*g* (*brakes off*). Red blood cells and other plasma constituents pellet to the bottom, while the heavier PBMC form a yellowish-coloured layer ('buffy coat') at the interface of the Ficoll-PBS/plasma gradient.
6. Remove PBMC by careful pipetting (use a small pipet, e.g., 5 mL), and transfer to a 15-mL tube.
7. Add warm PBS at a ratio of 1:4 (v/v), and centrifuge at 250*g* for 10 min (*brakes on*).
8. Wash pelleted cells by re-suspending in warm PBS and repeat. Repeated washes increase cell purity but decrease yield.
9. Resuspend PBMC in culture medium (we use T84 media for co-culture experiments), count and adjust to the desired cell density (we have used 10^6 cells/mL).

3.2.2. Lamina Propria Mononuclear Cell Isolation (Adapted from **ref. 17**).

For rodent cells, shave the animals' abdomen, wipe with ethanol, excise the desired section of intestine and flush away contents with warm (37°C) PBS; for human tissue, adherent material on the resected tissue is rinsed away with warm saline.

1. Place the tissue on filter paper, open along the mesenteric border, and place ~5 cm pieces into 100-mm culture plates containing warm culture media (supplemented with 1 m*M* dithiothreitol [DTT], a mucolytic agent) for 3 min.
2. Rinse with T84 media (or other suitable medium).
3. Transfer the tissue to fresh Petri dishes containing Hank's balanced salt solution (HBSS) with 130 μ*M* EDTA and incubate at 37°C for 15 min: this results in epithelial cell detachment.

4. Rinse twice with media to remove unwanted epithelial cells and any remaining mucus.
5. Scrape the mucosa from the muscle layer using a pair of glass slides.
6. Place the mucosa/submucosal scraping into 20 mL of medium supplemented with 20 U/mL collagenase and incubate at 37°C for 15 min.
7. Recover tissue, press through a wire-mesh screen (use a plunger from a sterile 10-mL syringe), and spin in a 50-mL tube at 200*g* for 10 min.
8. Discard the supernatant, and resuspend the pellet in 35 mL of 40% (v/v) media:iso-osmotic Percoll.
9. Underlay this solution with 15 mL 70% (v/v in media) iso-osmotic Percoll (*see* **Fig. 2**) using a Pasteur pipet.
10. Spin at 600*g* for 30 min with the *brakes off.*
11. Recover the cells by careful pipetting—the yellowish-colored 'buffy coat' layer at the Percoll interface contains the LPMC.
12. Add 20 mL culture media and spin at 250*g* for 10 min (*brakes on*).
13. Resuspend the pellet in 1 mL of media, and count cells using the trypan blue dye exclusion technique and resuspend cells at the desired concentration in a culture medium appropriate for the subsequent study (*see* **Note 7**).

3.2.3. Purification of PBMC or LPMC Subpopulations

Having obtained PBMC and LPMC, these mixed immune cell populations can be further purified to obtain: 1) T and B cells (i.e., monocyte/macrophage depleted), 2) T cells or B cells and subpopulations thereof based on surface markers (i.e., CD molecules), or 3) monocytes/macrophages only. Depletion of, or enrichment for, monocytes is most easily accomplished by plating PBMC in culture dishes and incubating at 37°C for at least 4 h (*see* **Note 11**); the nonadherent cells are collected as a source of T and B cells. To increase the yield, add ~5 mL warm PBS or culture media to the dish, swirl, and gently remove the supernatant. Dishes can now be discarded or used as a source of monocytes. Adherent cells can be gently scraped (with a cell scraper, rinsed first in 70% ethanol and then in sterile PBS) in a small volume of culture medium, which is then collected and spun at 250*g* for 10 min (*see* **Note 12**). Alternatively, to avoid scraping, PBMC or LPMC can be plated at the

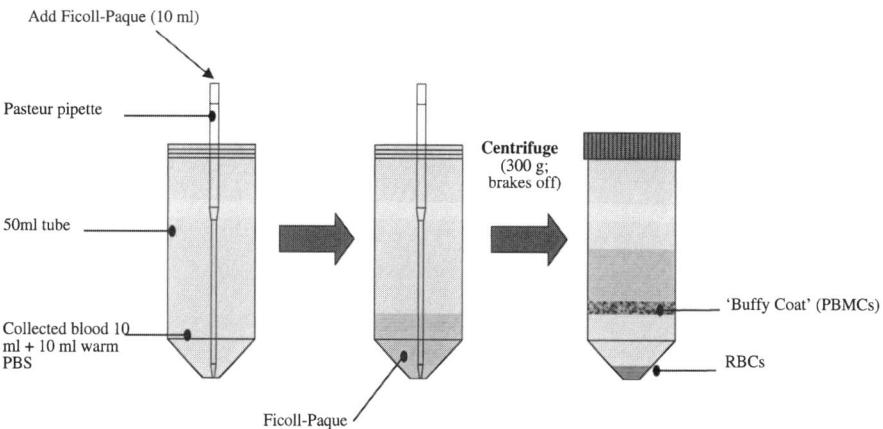

Fig. 2. Diagram of the procedural steps involved in PBMC isolation, focusing on creation of the Ficoll-Paque gradient and the resultant separation of the "buffy coat" (mononuclear cells) from the red blood cells and other plasma components.

desired density directly in the basal chamber of the co-culture plate and after 4 h incubation the medium is removed, the chamber rinsed with medium, leaving a relatively pure monocyte population (*see* **Notes 12** and **13**). Purified B cells or T cells are most easily acquired through positive or negative selection using immunomagnetic beads with monoclonal antibodies (MAbs) that react with cell-specific surface antigens (MACS; Miltenyl Biotec, Auburn, CA: see manufactures instructions). For additional cell-purification techniques the reader is referred to Current Protocols in Immunology *(17)*.

3.2.4. Cell Lines

An additional option is the use of cultured cell lines (e.g., Jurkat T cells, Ba/F3 B cells, Raw267.4 macrophages, etc.). We have used the human monocyte cell line THP-1 in place of PBMC. THP-1 cells grow in suspension; however, incubation with 10 nM 12-phorbol-13-myristic acid (PMA) for 2 d induces a macrophage-like phenotype and adherence to plastic (or glass) (*see* **Note 12**).

3.3. Immune Cell Activation and Epithelium Treatment

Two options are available to the researcher: incubating isolated immune cells with SAg in the basal chamber of transwells containing filter-grown epithelial monolayers (i.e., co-culture), or activating the immune cells separately and collecting the 'conditioned medium' (CM) for use in subsequent transwell experiments.

1. Fill (1.5 mL) the wells of a sterile 12-well plate with fresh medium (controls) or medium containing the desired concentration of immune cells.
2. Once the 12-well plate is prepared transfer in confluent filter-grown epithelial monolayers, thus establishing the co-culture.
3. Immune cells are then activated by addition of SAg (e.g., SEB at 1 μg/10^6 immune cells) to the basal compartment of the co-culture well.

Transepithelial resistance can be monitored throughout the co-culture period (*see* below: assessment of barrier function). At the end of the co-culture, the filter-grown epithelium can be used to assess the impact of superantigen-activated immune cells on ion transport (*see* **Subheading 3.5.**). Additionally, epithelia can be processed for examination by electron microscoproscopy, immunocytochemistry/immunocytoflourescence, Western blot, and any other standard cellular, molecular, or enzymatic assays.

As a modification of this approach, the immune cells can be activated in the absence of the epithelium and the CM collected and applied to the basal or apical compartment of culture wells containing naïve epithelial monolayers. Twenty-four hours after exposure of immune cells to SAg, the CM medium is collected, centrifuged at 200g for 10 min (to remove cells) and then used or stored at –20°C. (Note: avoid use of repeatedly freeze-thawed CM.) Use of CM offers some advantages over direct epithelial-immune cell co-culture experiments: 1) a single CM can be used for each epithelial monolayer in a transwell plate, reducing the variability that can be introduced to the experiment due to immune cell plating/growth; 2) when measuring the amounts of soluble mediators (e.g., cytokines) by enzyme-linked immunosorbent assay (ELISA), it is only necessary to use a sample from the CM and not from each individual transwell; 3) dose- and time-responses are simple experiments; 4) by separating the immune cells from the epithelium, different pharmacological treatments can be applied to each cell type (e.g., immune cells can be treated with steroids, then activated by SEB and the ability of this CM to affect epithelial function compared with CM collected from immune cells (from the same donor) that were not exposed to steroids *[18]*); 6) if assessing signal-transduction events, use of CM reduces the time response window by removing the time it takes (in co-culture) for newly activated immune cells to synthesize and release mediators. As a caveat it should be noted that use of immune cell populations in co-culture experiments can be considered a better recapitulation of the gut environment, allowing for cell–cell interactions and epithelial-immune cell cross-talk where the activity of the epithelium (e.g., mediator release) has the potential to modulate the immune response.

Finally, the length of culture will be determined by the experimental readout. For example, we see a characteristic drop in T84 transepithelial resistance (TER) and altered ion secretion after ~3–8 h of exposure to CM and after ~12 h in immune cell-epithelial co-cultures. Gene- and protein-expression events may be studied on a shorter time frame (e.g., 0.5–4 h) *(19)*, while signal transduction events may require culture with CM for only a few minutes *(20)*.

3.4. Role of the Epithelium

It is possible to investigate how the epithelium itself responds to culture with SEB-activated immune cells or CM by treatment with an inhibitory agent (e.g., steroids *(18)*, or inhibitors of specific intracellular signaling molecules *[21]*). Here the agent is added directly to the transwell, usually basally (*see* **Note 14**), before, at, or following exposure to CM or co-culture. This technique has allowed us to begin characterizing epithelial signaling events important in inflammatory mediator-induced changes to monolayer barrier function and ion secretion *(20,21)*.

3.5. Assessment of Epithelial Ion Transport

3.5.1. Assessing Epithelial Ion Transport with Ussing Chambers

At the outset, it must be emphasized that only those cell lines that establish stable polarized monolayers with functional tight junctions are suitable for the following analyses (*see* **Note 1**).

The study of vectorial ion transport and barrier function is readily accomplished via use of the Ussing chamber (*22, see* **Fig. 3**). The epithelial monolayer (on filter supports) is mounted between joining halves of the leucite chamber, both serosally and mucosally bathed by identical pre-oxygenated physiological buffers that nullify any hydrostatic or chemi-osmotic gradients. A variety of buffers are available for use; we use Kreb's buffer supplemented with 10 m*M* glucose (*see* **Notes 15** and **16**). Each chamber half has two ports for agar bridges, which are connected via a reservoir of saturated KCl to either calomel reference electrodes or silver/silver chloride electrodes for measuring potential difference and injecting current, respectively. The pair of bridges placed closest to the epithelium serve to monitor the spontaneous potential difference generated by the cells, while the bridges that are more distant from the epithelium are used for the injection of current (*see* **Fig. 3**). The chambers are oxygenated by a gas-lift and maintained at ~37°C by a heated water circulatory system. In the voltage-clamp setting, the potential difference (PD) across the epithelium is maintained at 0 volts, and the current that must be injected to maintain the 0 voltage is the short-circuit current, or Isc (in $\mu A/cm^2$). Current is injected in response to active ion-transport events, and thus, the Isc is reflective of the net charge movement across the monolayer. It should be remembered that electrolyte transport creates the driving force for directed water movement, which, in the intestine, can result in a diarrheal response or constipation. It should also be noted that the Isc indicates net charge movement but does not reveal the identity of the charge carrying ion (*see* **Note 17**).

In addition to continuous monitoring of baseline (or tonic) Isc, stimulated Isc responses can be assessed by recording the peak change in Isc, or area under the curve, in response to pro-secretory (e.g.,

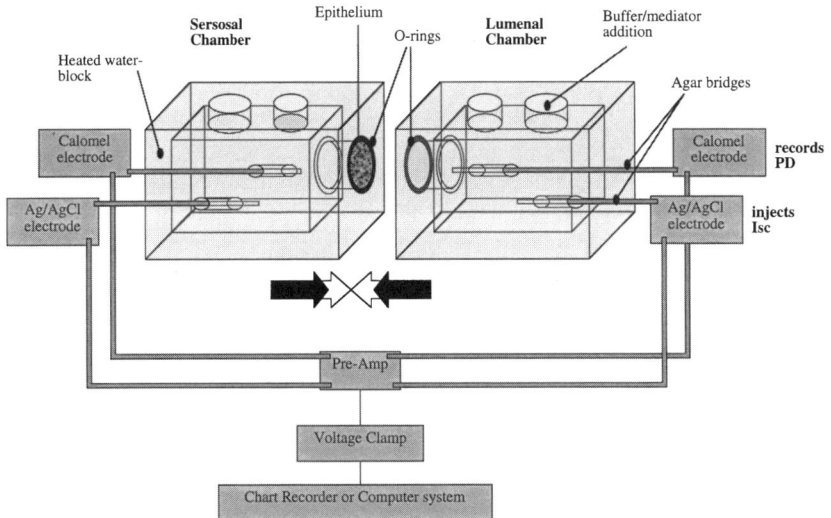

Fig. 3. Diagram of the Ussing chamber apparatus, designed to accept filter-grown epithelial monolayers. The buffer reservoirs (luminal and serosal) are maintained at 37°C by a surrounding heated water-jacket; buffers are mixed and aerated by gas-lifts (not shown). PD, potential difference; Isc, short-circuit current.

forskolin [Fsk], cholera toxin) or pro-absorptive (e.g., neuropeptide Y [NPY]) agents added directly into the appropriate side of the Ussing chamber. The Isc responsiveness can be presented as $\mu A/cm^2$ (*see* **Fig. 4**). Alternatively, because there can be variability between cell passages, the data can normalized to time-matched naïve epithelial monolayer responses and presented as percent of control events.

3.5.2. Assessing Epithelial Ion Transport Using Voltmeter and Chopstick Electrodes

In the absence of the Ussing chamber-voltage clamp apparatus a calculated Isc can be obtained using a voltmeter and chopstick electrodes and taking readings directly from the transwell plate.

1. The electrodes must be equilibrated by selecting voltage on the voltmeter and placing the electrodes in the buffer of choice for 1 h.
2. Prepare a 12-well plate as follows: the top row wells contain Kreb's + glucose, the middle row Kreb's buffer + 0.01 M Fsk, and the bot-

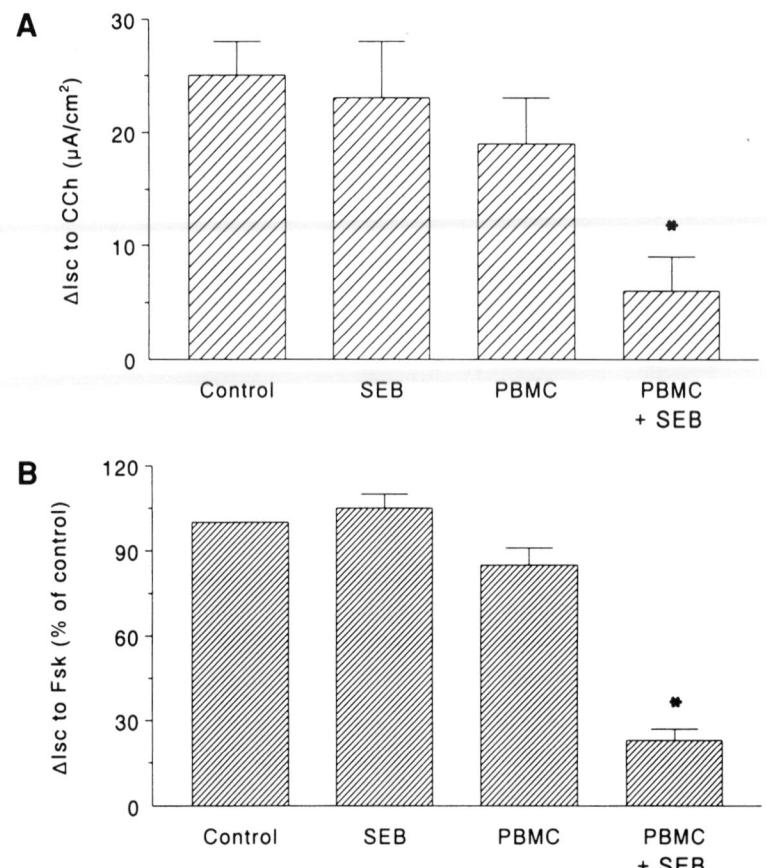

Fig. 4. Bar charts showing the (**A**) the change in short-circuit current
(ΔIsc) evoked by carbachol (CCh, 10^{-4} M; presented as units of current)
and (**B**) in response to forskolin (Fsk, 10^{-5} M; presented as a percentage
of the control monolayer response) in T84 monolayers that had been
co-cultured with peripheral blood mononuclear cells (PBMC, 10^6 cells) $\pm$
Staphylococcus aureus enterotoxin B (SEB, 1 µg/mL) for 48 h and then
mounted in Ussing chambers ($n = 6$–12 epithelial monolayers; *, $p < 0.05$
compared to control). Original data adapted from **ref.** *(10)*.

tom row Kreb's + 0.1 M carbachol (CCh) (*see* **Fig. 5**) (Fsk and CCh
allow assessment of Cl^- secretion in response to cAMP and Ca^{2+}
mobilization, respectively *[10]*) One 12-well plate so prepared is
used for 4 epithelial monolayers.

3. Place the 12-well plate on a heating pad and allow to warm.

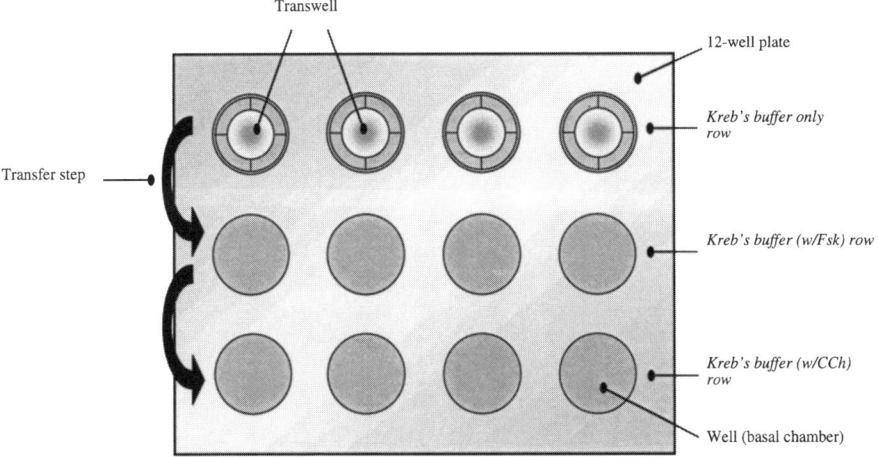

Fig. 5. Diagram showing 12-well plate set-up for determining the calculated short-circuit current (Isc) as determined by changes in potential difference and transepithelial resistance in response to the adenylate cyclase activator, forskolin (Fsk) and subsequently the cholinergic agonist carbachol (CCh) using the Millipore voltmeter and chopstick electrodes.

4. Aspirate apical and basal media from the transwells to be tested (maximum 4 at a time) and add Kreb's buffer to the apical compartment.

5. To equilibrate the monolayer, transwells are transferred to the top row of the prepared 12-well plate and voltage and resistance values are recorded at time 0 and 5 min later. It is critical the voltmeter be set to read resistance while electrodes are being transferred between wells (or at anytime when they are not in buffer).

6. Take readings again after 10 min, the voltage reading should be steady before continuing with the experiment.

7. Transfer all transwells to the middle row containing the Fsk and record voltage and resistance at 5 min intervals until a peak response is determined (*see* **Note 18**).

8. Next move only 2 wells at a time (*see* **Note 19**) into the CCh solution and record voltage and resistance every 30 s for 4 min until the peak response has been surpassed.

9. Repeat for the remaining 2 epithelial monolayers.

To calculate Isc apply Ohm's Law:

$$\text{Voltage (V)} = \text{Current (I)} \times \text{Resistance (R)}$$

3.6. Assessing Barrier Properties

3.6.1. Transepithelial Electrical Resistance (TER)

TER indicates the passive flux of ions across the preparation and is generally considered a reflection of the leakiness of the tight junctions. Monolayers are mounted in the Ussing chamber and the voltage clamp is set in the bipolar mode, which allows the voltage to be jumped from 0 volts to, for example, 1 milli-volt at pre-set intervals. The change in Isc that occurs in response to 1 mV change in potential difference allows for the calculation of resistance via the Ohmic relationship. This procedure is referred to as the differential pulse technique and is the most sensitive measure of TER (*see* **Fig. 6**).

Alternatively, the Millopore voltmeter and chopstick electrodes are an inexpensive and convenient means to monitor TER. This simple procedure, although slightly less sensitive than the Ussing chamber, confers two advantages to the investigator: first, TER can be monitored daily under sterile conditions so that the investigator can define when epithelial preparations are suitable for experimentation, e.g., TER ≥ 800 Ω/cm^2; and second, paired analyses can be performed since TER can be monitored before and after co-culture with SAg-activated immune cells or exposure to CM (*see* **Fig.6**).

3.6.2. Small-Molecule Flux

In addition to TER, epithelial barrier function should be assessed by monitoring the flux of "marker" molecules that are radiolabeled (e.g., ^{51}Cr-EDTA), fluorescently labeled (e.g., dextrans; Molecular Probes, Eugene, OR) or have an associated assayable enzymatic activity (e.g., horseradish peroxidase). Flux experiments can be performed when the epithelium is mounted in the Ussing chamber (*see* **Note 20**) or in transwell plates. The study of barrier function is often accomplished using ^{51}Cr-EDTA, ^{3}H-mannitol or ^{3}H-inulin—all small molecules that primarily cross the epithelium via the paracellular pathway. The probe molecule is added to either the basolateral (serosal) or apical (lumenal) compartment (now the "hot" side) and

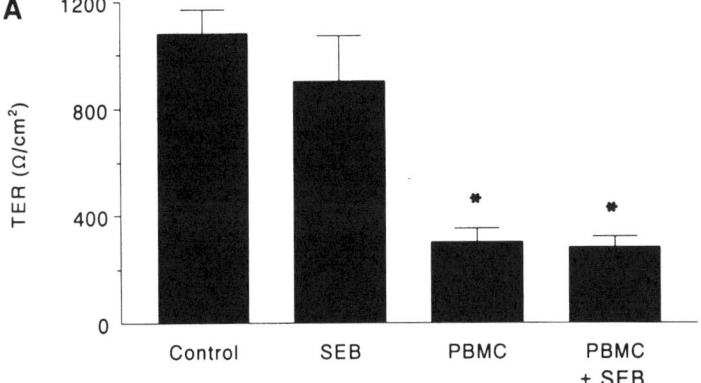

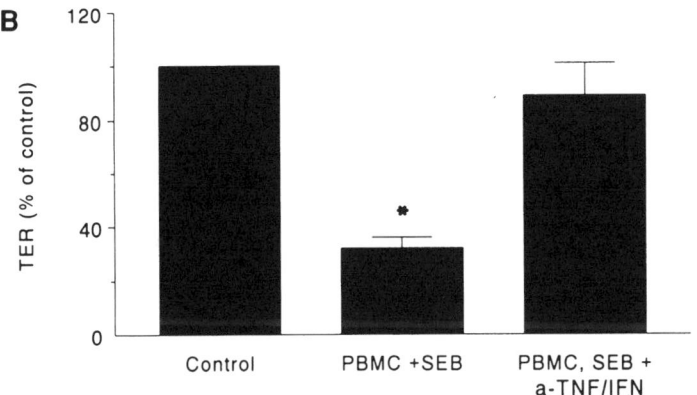

Fig. 6. Bar charts showing the **(A)** the change in transepithelial resistance (TER) in T84 monolayers that had been co-cultured with peripheral blood mononuclear cells (PBMC, 10^6 cells) ± *Staphylococcus aureus* enterotoxin B (SEB, 1 µg/mL) for 48 h and **(B)** the effect of including neutralizing antibodies against tumor necrosis factor-α (TNF-α) and interferon-γ (IFN-γ) (1–5 µg/mL) on PBMC+SEB induced changes in TER (presented as a percentage of control, where control TER ranged from 1000–1545 $\Omega.cm^2$) (n = 6–12 epithelial monolayers; *, $p < 0.05$ compared to control). Original data adapted from **ref. *(10)*.**

any potential osmotic effects countered by adding an equal volume (at the same concentration) of the nonlabeled probe to the "cold" side.

1. Epithelial monolayers are mounted in the Ussing chambers and allowed to establish a stable Isc and TER (~10–15 min).

2. The probe (e.g., 6.5 µCi ^{3}H-mannitol *[13]*) is added to the luminal buffer and allowed to equilibrate for 30 min.

3. Samples (500 µL) are taken from the cold side at 20- or 30-min intervals (and replaced with the appropriate cold buffer) over a 90-min period.

4. Samples (50 µL) are taken from the hot side at the beginning and end of the experiment to calculate probe-specific activity.

5. Radioactivity is determined by counting in a γ- or scintillation counter (*see* **Note 21**) and the flux presented as: 1) counts (or degradations) per minute (cpm); 2) percent cpm crossing the monolayer compared to initial cpm on the hot side; 3) flux rates calculated in amount.h.cm^2 by standard formulae *(22)*; or 4) in the case of ionic fluxes, converted to µEquivalents.h.cm^2.

Clearly, increased transepithelial flux of the probe indicates increased epithelial permeability (*see* **Fig. 7**).

3.7. Conclusions

Recognizing the potency of SAg as T-cell activating agents, one would intuitively accept that these bacterial products could play an important role in initiating or aggravating inflammatory or autoimmune diseases. The complexity of a dynamic multi-functional tissue such as the gut means that the interpretation of in vivo, and indeed ex vivo tissue, studies are hampered by the fact that many intercellular communications can converge to influence a single physiological/pathophysiological event. To this end, the use of filter-grown epithelial monolayers in vitro has enabled precise assessment of SAg-immune activation on epithelial electrolyte transport and permeability, and as such has facilitated the growing awareness that immune cells and their products (e.g., cytokines) influence the physiological processes of the intestinal epithelium.

4. Notes

1. The human T84 cell line has features characteristic of colonic crypt-like epithelial cells including polarization, secretagogue-induced chloride secretion and the formation of tight junctions (can have extremely high TER, 1000–4000 Ω/cm^2) and so are often favored

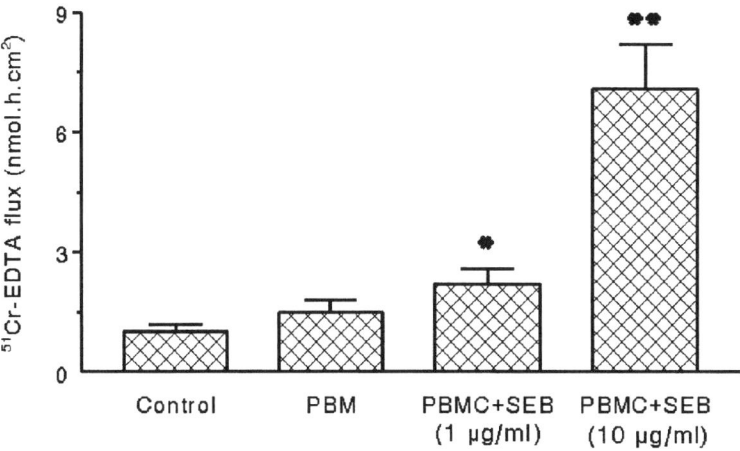

Fig. 7. Bar chart showing the increase in transepithelial flux of the inert marker of paracellular permeability, ^{51}Cr-EDTA, across T84 monolayers that had been co-cultured with peripheral blood mononuclear cells (PBMC, 10^6 cells) ± *Staphylococcus aureus* enterotoxin B (SEB) for 48 h and then mounted in Ussing chambers ($n = 3$–8 epithelial monolayers; * and **, $p < 0.05$ compared to control and PBMC + SEB at 1 μg/mL). Original data adapted from **ref. (10)**.

for the study of vectorial ion transport and paracellular permeability. The HT-29 and CaCo-2 human gut epithelial cell lines are of similar value in assessing ion transport and barrier function, although their baseline TER seldom exceeds 500 Ω/cm^2. Also, by varying the culture conditions CaCo-2 cells can be induced to differentiate from a crypt-like cell to a villus-like cell (23). If ion transport and permeability are not the focus of interest, then other epithelia can be employed. For example, rodent epithelial cell lines (IEC-6, IEC-18, KATO III) offer the advantage that they can be co-cultured with LPMC obtained from mice with any number of experimentally induced enteropathies.

2. PBMC populations isolated from donor blood vary in cell number and subtype, but generally yield at least 10^6 cells/mL blood, consisting of ~70–75% T cells, ~10–15% B cells and ~5–10% monocytes.

3. The final media recipe is determined by the cell type being cultured and will be provided with the cell line. Alternatively, recipes for many types of cell-culture medium are available from the ATCC website at http://www.atcc.org.

4. A transwell—or "filter support"—consists of a well and a plastic insert that rests above the bottom of the well (*see* **Fig. 1**). The base of the insert is a porous filter upon which cells are cultured. In this manner, independent access is granted to the apical (mucosal/luminal) and basal (serosal/basolateral) sides of the epithelium. Different transwells are available, including a clear (polyester) filter if visualization of cells on the filter is important, and transwells with pore sizes ranging from 0.1–12 μm. Transwells can be purchased in different sizes, including 6-, 12-, and 24-well plates, with the size of the filter diminishing as number per plate increases. As a modification of this monolayer orientation, the transwells can be placed in small sterile beakers, inverted and epithelial cells seeded onto the bottom (or outside) of the filter. Eight hours later, the transwells are returned to the culture plate in their correct orientation, effectively having the luminal side of the growing monolayer facing the bottom of the culture well (*see* **Fig. 1**). In this orientation, immune cells (e.g., neutrophils) can be added into the transwell, juxtaposing them to the basal surface of the enterocytes and facilitating transepithelial migration studies in response to chemotactic substances placed in the basal compartment of the culture well *(24)*.

5. Passage cells by standard methods. We follow a PBS (warm, sterile) rinse with incubation (37°C, 10–45 min) in 6–8 mL 0.25% trypsin-EDTA. Upon detachment, 12 mL T84 medium is added, cells are collected in a sterile 50-mL tube, centrifuged at 50g for 5 min and resuspended in 20 mL medium.

6. Confluence is determined by viewing at high magnification. A flask in which all individual cells are making contact with no obvious "holes" in the monolayer is said to be fully confluent. In cell culture, it is generally advised that cells not be allowed to reach full confluence, and if at confluence, should be split. For example, T84 and HT-29 cells are highly adherent and grow slowly, whereas CaCo-2 cells begin detaching upon reaching confluence.

7. Mix 50 μL of the cell suspension (*see* **Note 5**) with 150 μL 0.04% trypan blue dye (dead cells stain blue) and count the viable (nonstained) cells on a haemocytometer. By counting the cells in the 4 large squares on the haemocytometer slide (i.e., those delineated by triple lines), the investigator has accounted for the 1:4 dilution in the trypan blue solution and can multiply the count by 10^5 to calculate the number of cells/mL in the original solution.

8. Other investigators have seeded T84 cells at lower densities (i.e., 2.5–5×10^5 cells/filter) and have found the resultant monolayers suitable for use in Ussing chamber studies.

9. If using T84 cells the investigator must define what a control monolayer is. Usually this is a minimum TER (e.g., $\geq 800\ \Omega/cm^2$).

10. Shake Ficoll-Paque well before use, draw 10 mL into a syringe and inject via large-bore needle into the Pasteur pipet.

11. It has been reported that the presence of serum increases the time for monocyte adherence. Thus, if the original PBMC isolates are suspended in serum-free media, it is possible to reduce plating time ~1 h *(17)*.

12. Exploiting the ability of monocytes to adhere to plastic or glass is a simple and inexpensive method of gross purification. However, it has been noted that anchorage promotes a macrophage-like phenotype, and, as an activation stimulus, can induce gene transcription and protein expression *(25)*. In light of this, when using monocytes in co-culture experiments we allow a 24 h "resting" period after adherence before incubation with epithelial cells or any further treatments.

13. The guidelines in this section are generalizations and are reasonable starting points in co-culture experiments. However, it is essential that mixed immune cell populations be fully characterized by differential staining and/or fluorescent-activated cell sorting (FACS) analysis.

14. Generally we add inhibitors and other agents (cytokines, etc.) to the basal well due to the polarized basolateral expression of receptors on intestinal epithelia; however, it is physiologically relevant to add other stimuli (e.g., bacterial products) to the apical compartment.

15. Owing to the luminal expression of a Na^+-glucose cotransporter, if using small intestinal epithelial cells, mannitol rather then glucose should be used in the luminal buffer as glucose will drive Na^+ transport and increase the Isc.

16. Just prior to use, the buffer should be warmed and oxygenated (~10 min) and then adjusted such that the pH is between 7.33–7.37.

17. A number of strategies can be employed to identify the ionic species responsible for changes in Isc. Ussing chamber studies can be conducted with bathing buffers in which specific ions have been removed and replaced with a similarly charged ion, to maintain the electrical balance (e.g. Cl^--free buffers *[26]*). Also, experiments can be conducted in the presence of specific pharmacological blockers

of ion channels or pumps (e.g., Cl⁻ or Na⁺ channel blockers (i.e., amiloride, sodium channel blocker), inhibitors of the Na⁺/K⁺/2Cl⁻ co-transporter [i.e., bumetinide], etc.). By using radiolabeled ions such as $^{36}Cl^-$ (or ^{125}I), ^{22}Na, or ^{86}Rb and conducting bidirectional flux studies one can unequivocally define the role of chloride, sodium and potassium movements in any Isc change, respectively *(22)*.

18. T84 cells display a rapid and prolonged response to Fsk. If using other cell types the time interval between potential difference and resistance readings may have to be adjusted to determine the peak Isc response.

19. T84 cells respond almost instantaneously to CCh, attempting the monitoring of more than two monolayers will result in missing the peak response in individual monolayers.

20. For flux experiments in Ussing chambers, it is critical that the experiment start with equal volumes on each side of the epithelial preparation and that this volume be maintained throughout the experiment. Loss of buffer caused by excessive bubbling or leaks from either buffer invalidates the data. Silicon grease can be used to seal any leaks during the initial equilibrium period prior to addition of the probe to the designated hot buffer.

21. Dual fluxes with γ- and β-emitter probes can be conducted (e.g., ^{51}Cr-EDTA and ^3H-mannitol, respectively *[10]*) but it must be remembered that the γ-emission will be detected in the scintillation counter. Thus a pure sample (2 or 3 dilutions) of the γ-emitter should be counted in the γ-counter and the scintillation counter so that a correction factor can be calculated to account for the percent of the cpm determined in the scintillation counter that is due to, in this example, ^{51}Cr-EDTA and not ^3H-mannitol.

Acknowledgments

Studies citied from the authors' laboratory were funded by operating grants from the Canadian Institutes for Health Research (MT-13421: formerly the Medical Research Council of Canada) and the Crohn's and Colitis Foundation of Canada.

References

1. McKay, D. M. and Perdue, M. H. (1993) Intestinal epithelial function: the case for immunophysiological regulation. Cells and mediators (first of two parts). *Dig. Dis. Sci.* **38,** 1377–1387.

2. Perdue, M. H. and McKay, D. M. (1994) Integrative immunophysiology in the intestinal mucosa. *Am. J. Physiol. (Gastrointest. Liver Physiol.)* **267,** G151–G165.

3. McKay, D. M. and Baird, A. W. (1999) Cytokine regulation of epithelial permeability and ion transport. *Gut* **44,** 283–289.

4. Berin, M. C., McKay, D. M., and Perdue, M. H. (1999) Immune-epithelial interactions in host defense. *Am. J. Trop. Med. Hyg.* **60(4 Suppl.),** 16–25.

5. Philpott, D. J., McKay, D. M., Sherman, P. M., and Perdue, M. H. (1996) Infection of T84 cells with enteropathogenic *Escherichia coli* alters barrier and transport functions. *Am. J. Physiol. (Gastrointest. Liver Physiol.)* **270,** G634–G645.

6. McKay, D. M. (1999) Intestinal inflammation and the gut microflora. *Can. J. Gastroenterol.* **13,** 509–516.

7. Fraser, J., Arcus, V., Kong, P., Baker, E., and Proft, T. (2000) Superantigens: powerful modifiers of the immune system. *Mol. Med. Today* **3,** 125–132.

8. McKay, D. M., Benjamin, M. A., and Lu, J. (1998) CD4⁺ T cells mediate superantigen-induced abnormalities in murine jejunal ion transport. *Am. J. Physiol. (Gastrointest. Liver Physiol.)* **275,** G29–G38.

9. Benjamin, M. A., Lu, J., Donnelly, G., Dureja, P., and McKay D. M. (1998) Changes in murine jejunal morphology evoked by the bacterial superantigen *Staphylococcus aureus* entertoxin B are mediated by CD4⁺ T cells. *Infect. Immunity* **66,** 2193–2199.

10. McKay, D. M. and Singh, P. K. (1997) Superantigen activation of immune cells evokes epithelial (T84) transport and barrier abnormalities via IFN-γ and TNFα: inhibition of increased permeability, but not diminished secretory responses by TGF-β₂. *J. Immunol.* **159,** 2382–2390.

11. Donnelly, G. A. E., Lu, J., Takeda, T., and McKay D. M. (1999) Colonic epithelial physiology is altered in response to the bacterial superantigen *Yersinia pseudotuberculosis* mitogen. *J. Infect. Dis.* **180,** 1590–1596.

12. Lu, J., Philpott, D. J., Saunders, P. R., Perdue, M. H., Yang, P.-C., and McKay D. M. (1998) Epithelial ion transport abnormalities evoked by superantigen-activated immune cells are inhibited by interleukin-10 but not interleukin-4. *J. Pharmacol. Exp. Ther.* **287,** 128–136.

13. McKay, D. M., Croitoru, K., and Perdue, M. H. (1996) T cell-monocyte interactions regulate epithelial physiology in a coculture model of inflammation. *Am J. Physiol. (Cell Physiol.)* **270,** C419–C428.

14. McKay, D. M., Philpott, D. J., and Perdue, M. H. (1997) Review article: in vitro models in inflammatory bowel disease research: a critical review. *Aliment. Pharmacol. Ther.* **11(Suppl. 3),** 70–80.

15. Panja, A. (2000) A novel method for the establishment of a pure population of non-transformed human intestinal primary epithelial cell (HIPEC) lines in long term culture. *Lab. Invest.* **80,** 1473–1475.

16. Pang, G., Buret, A., O'Loughlin, E., Smith, A., Batey, R., and Clancy, R. (1996) Immunologic, functional, and morphological characterization of three new human small intestinal epithelial cell lines. *Gastroenterology* **111,** 8–18.

17. Unit 7.6: (2001) Isolation of monocyte/macrophage populations. In: *Current Protocols in Immunology*, vol. 2 (Colgan, J. E. et al., eds.) John Wiley and Sons Inc., New York, NY, pp. 7.6.1–7.6.8

18. McKay, D. M., Brattsand, R., Wieslander, E., Fung, M., Croitoru, K., and Perdue, M. H. (1996) Budesonide inhibits T cell initiated epithelial pathophysiology in an *in vitro* model of inflammation. *J. Pharm. Exp. Ther.* **277,** 403–410.

19. Jedrzkiewicz, S., Kataeva, G., Hogaboam, C. M., Kunkel, S. L., Strieter, R. M., and McKay, D. M. (1999) Superantigen immune stimulation evokes epithelial monocyte chemoattractant protein 1 and RANTES production. *Infect. Immunity* **67,** 6198–6202.

20. McKay, D. M., Botelho, F., Ceponis, P. J., and Richards, C. D. (2000) Superantigen immune stimulation activates epithelial STAT-1 and PI 3-K: PI 3-K regulation of permeability. *Am. J. Physiol. (Gastrointest. Liver Physiol.)* **279,** G1094–G1103.

21. Ceponis, P. J., Botelho, F., Richards, C. D., and McKay, D. M. (2000) Interleukins 4 and 13 increase intestinal epithelial permeability by a phosphatidylinositol 3-kinase pathway: lack of evidence for STAT 6. *J. Biol. Chem.* **275,** 29,132–29,137.

22. Karnaky, K. J., Jr. (1992) Electrophysiological assessment of epithelia, in *Cell-Cell Interactions: A Practical Approach* (Stevenson, B.

R. Gallin, W. J. and Paul, D. L., eds.), IRL Press at Oxford University Press, Oxford, UK, pp. 257–273.

23. Abraham, C., Scaglione-Sewell, B., Skaroski, S. F., Qin, W., Bissonnette, M., and Brasitius, T. A. (1998) Protein kinase Cα modulates growth and differentiation in Caco2 cells. *Gasteroenterology* **114,** 503–509.

24. Madara, J. L., Colgan, S., Nusrat, A., Delp, C., and Parkos, C. (1992) A simple approach to measurement of electrical parameters of cultured epithelial monolayers: use in assessing neutrophil-epithelial interactions. *J. Tiss. Cult. Methods* **14,** 209–216.

25. Haskill, S., Johnson, C., Eierman, D., Becker, S., and Warren, K. (1988) Adherence induces selective mRNA expression of monocyte mediators and proto-oncogenes. *J. Immunol.* **140,** 1690–1694.

26. Saunders, P. R., Kosecka, U., McKay, D. M., and Perdue, M. H. (1994) Acute stressors stimulate ion secretion and increase epithelial permeability in the rat intestine. *Am. J. Physiol. (Gastrointest. Liver Phsiol.)* **267,** G794–G799.

15

Pyrogenic, Lethal, and Emetic Properties of Superantigens in Rabbits and Primates

John K. McCormick, Gregory A. Bohach,
and Patrick M. Schlievert

1. Introduction

Superantigens (SAgs) stimulate large fractions of T cells by circumventing normal antigen presentation through binding both class II major histocompatibility complex (MHC) molecules on antigen-presenting cells, and specific variable regions on the β-chain (V_β) of the T-cell antigen receptor (TCR) *(1,2)*. The bacterial SAgs produced from coagulase positive staphylococci (*Staphylococcus aureus*) and group A streptococci (GAS; *Streptococcus pyogenes*) belong to the large and expanding family of pyrogenic toxins, and various members of this group of SAgs have a clear involvement in the toxic shock syndrome (TSS). Through SAg-mediated stimulation, T lymphocytes are activated at several orders of magnitude above antigen-specific activation, resulting in the extensive release of cytokines that are believed to be responsible for the most severe features of TSS. SAgs from *S. aureus* include toxic shock syndrome toxin-1 (TSST-1), multiple staphylococcal enterotoxin (SE) serotypes (A through P, excluding F), while SAgs from *S. pyogenes* include streptococcal pyrogenic exotoxin (SPE) serotypes (A, C, G,

From: *Methods in Molecular Biology, vol. 214: Superantigen Protocols*
Edited by: T. Krakauer © Humana Press Inc., Totowa, NJ

H, I, J) as well as streptococcal superantigen (SSA) and multiple streptococcal mitogenic exotoxin Z (SMEZ) variants *(3–5)*. The toxins within this class of SAgs that have been tested are all pyrogenic, and all are likely to be capable to induce TSS in susceptible hosts if supplied in sufficient quantity.

Other than superantigenicity, in vivo animal models have generally been used for the study of the major biological effects of the bacterial SAgs. These activities include determination of both pyrogenic (fever induction) and toxic (lethal and emetic) activities. Although most studies on the lethal effects of the SAgs have been conducted in mice, we believe this animal model may not be appropriate because mice are generally very resistant to the lethal effects of these toxins *(6)*. In fact, most mouse strains do not develop a disease resembling TSS even after high dose of SAg alone by injection, or through continuous infusion. Sensitizing agents are commonly used, such as the hepatotoxin D-galactosamine, which renders mice susceptible to SAg induced lethal activity and results in the development of fulminant liver failure, which may be caused by extensive tumor necrosis factor-α (TNF-α) mediated hepatocellular apoptosis *(7–9)*. However, a similar condition has not been reported in patients with clinical TSS and this discrepancy has raised important questions regarding the validity of mouse models of TSS *(4,6)*. Although rabbits are also resistant to toxic affects of SAgs when administered as an intravenous bolus, we believe this animal is a more appropriate model of toxicity because rabbits develop a lethal disease that is similar to TSS when low doses of SAg are administered by means of continuous infusion *(10)*. The SEs also show toxicity as the agents of staphylococcal food-borne illness by inducing emesis when ingested orally, although this activity is restricted to the SEs and is not shared with the streptococcal SAgs or TSST-1.

In this chapter, we will focus on the methods used to determine pyrogenic and toxic (lethal shock) activity of the bacterial SAgs in rabbits, as well as emetic activity of the SEs in primates.

2. Materials

1. Phosphate-buffered saline (PBS): 5 mM Na$_2$HPO$_4$/NaH$_2$PO$_4$ buffer, 150 mM NaCl, at pH 7.2.
2. Superantigens (SAgs): It is necessary to obtain highly purified preparations of the SAg, often in significant quantity, to conduct these studies. Due to the potency of the SAgs, it is often desirable to obtain recombinant toxins expressed from *E. coli* to rule out interference of other SAgs expressed from the same host; however, preparations obtained from *E. coli* may be contaminated with endotoxin which is a major pyrogen. Purification of these proteins has been discussed elsewhere or commercial preparations can be obtained from Toxin Technologies, Sarasota, FL. All preparations must be dissolved in PBS, and not water, for biological activity determinations.
3. Endotoxin: It is necessary to obtain endotoxin preparations for the enhancement of endotoxin shock model of TSS. The gold standard for the isolation and preparation of endotoxin is generally considered to be the method by Westphal et al. *(11)* although this and other methods were recently reviewed *(12)*. For our experiments, we use endotoxin purified from *Salmonella enterica* serovar Typhimurium by the hot phenol method *(11)*.
4. Pyrogen free syringes and needles can be obtained from various sources. We use Monoject syringes and aluminum hub hypodermic needles (25- and 29-gauge) from Sherwood Medical Company (St. Louis, MO).
5. Miniosmotic pumps (Model 2001) are available from Alza Pharmaceuticals (Palo Alto, CA). These pumps are designed to release 1.0 µL of their contents (200 µL) per hour over a period of 7 d.
6. Pyrogen test rack for animal restraint and multiple rectal thermometer apparatus. Equipment must be approved for animal use and should be obtained through the institutional research animals resources.
7. Ketamine (100 mg/mL): (Phoenix Pharmaceuticals, Inc., St. Joseph, MO).
8. Xylazine (20 mg/mL): (Phoenix Pharmaceuticals, Inc.).
9. Sutures: We obtain our sutures from Sherwood Medical (3-0 Silk, CE-6 needle).
10. Euthanasia solution. Use a barbiturate solution approved at your institution. We use Beuthanasia-D special (active ingredients: 390 mg/

mL phentobarbital, 50 mg/mL phenytoin sodium), Schering-Plough
Animal Health (Union, NJ).

11. Sterile surgeon's blade can be obtained from various sources. We
    use Personna Plus Microcoat blades (No. 22) from the American
    Safety Razor Company (Staunton, VA).
12. Artificially flavored fruit punch (Lyons-Magnus, Clovis, CA).
13. Rabbits: Young adult American Dutch belted rabbits (1.5–2.0 kg)
    are typically used for the pyrogenicity and lethal studies. We obtain
    our rabbits from Birchwood Farms (Redwing, MN).
14. Monkeys: We use pigtail monkeys (*Macaca nemestrina*) for emesis
    studies although, if unavailable, other species of macaques (Rhesus
    and cynomolgus) have been used successfully. Young adult pigtail
    monkeys (up to 10 kilograms) generate reliable results and can be
    handled effectively for this assay.

3. Methods

The methods described in this chapter involve the use of live
experimental animals and all procedures must first be approved by
the institutions animal care committee or other appropriate regulatory agency. All investigators and staff must be properly trained to
perform animal experiments.

3.1. Pyrogenicity

This section describes the accepted method to determine pyrogenicity of the bacterial SAgs. In general, 3–5 American Dutch belted
rabbits are used per group to establish pyrogenic activity, and an
average increase of 0.5°C over 4 h is considered to be pyrogenic.
Positive controls can include any of the known pyrogenic toxin
SAgs such as TSST-1, SEB, SEC, SPE A, or SPE C. Negative controls consist of an equivalent volume of PBS administered via the
marginal ear vein in a separate group from the same cohort.

1. Install and acclimatize rabbits in the pyrogen test rack for 4 h 1 d
   prior to the actual pyrogenicity test. If animals are not acclimatized,
   variability between rabbits will be increased.
2. The following day, install rabbits in the pyrogen test rack and insert
   rectal thermocouples. After 60 min record baseline temperatures.

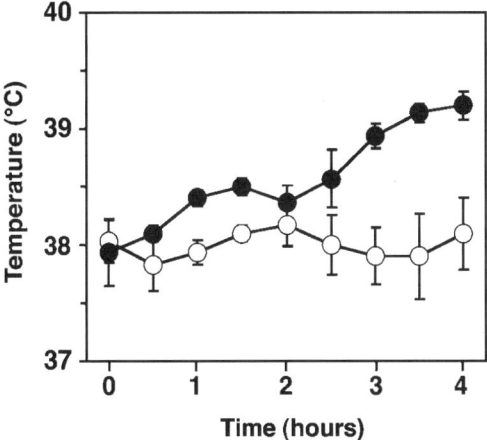

Fig. 1. Time-course temperature measurements of fever responses to 5 μg/kg of SPE A in PBS. Three rabbits per group were used and average temperatures ± standard errors (SEs) are shown for each time point. Five μg/mL of SPE A in PBS (*close circles*) and equivalent volume of PBS (*open circles*) are shown.

3. Rabbits are injected in the marginal ear vein with 5 μg of SAg per kg dissolved in PBS. We prepare our toxins in 5 μg/mL PBS solutions. Animals remain in the pyrogen test rack and temperatures are recorded at 4 h as above using the rectal thermocouples. A time-course experiment using 5 μg/mL of purified SPE A in PBS is shown in **Fig. 1** with a control group of rabbits that received the same volume of PBS.

4. We typically use the same cohort of rabbits to conduct experiments with the endotoxin enhancement model of TSS (*see* **Subheading 3.2.**) if this activity is to be determined.

3.2. Endotoxin Enhancement Model of Toxic Shock Syndrome

This section describes the model originally described by Kim and Watson *(13)* and Schlievert *(14)* to determine the ability of the bacterial SAgs to induce enhancement of susceptibility to endotoxin induced shock.

1. Either continue the pyrogenicity test in **Subheading 3.1.** or repeat

that method as described. If pyrogenicity is not to be determined, the animals do not require acclimatization nor do they need to be installed in the pyrogen test rack.

2. At 4 h following injection of the SAg, inject 10 µg/kg of endotoxin (approx 1/50 lethal dose) dissolved in PBS via the marginal ear vein. This can be done in the pyrogen test rack or in another approved restraining device.

3. Monitor animals for symptoms of TSS which can be defined as the absence of an escape response and the failure of the animals to right themselves. If these conditions present, our research animal use permit requires the animals be euthanized. Other conditions often include hyperventilation, diarrhea, and mottling of the faces.

4. Mortality, as defined by death or conditions of premature termination, is monitored for 48 h following injection of endotoxin.

5. If premature termination is required, or if the animal survives past the 48 h time point, euthanasia is achieved by placing the animal in the restraining device and administering (150 mg/kg of barbiturate IV via the marginal ear vein.

3.3. Miniosmotic Pump Model of Toxic Shock Syndrome

The miniosmotic pump model of TSS *(10)* has been used to establish toxic activity of various pyrogenic toxin SAgs. The model is generally considered as the more accepted model of TSS compared with the endotoxin enhancement model of TSS (*see* **Subheading 3.2.**). Miniosmotic pumps are used because they are designed to release a constant amount of product into the subcutaneous tissue over various times, which is similar to what would occur during infection with a toxigenic *S. aureus* or *S. pyogenes*. We typically use three to five rabbits for each toxin preparation to be tested.

1. Miniosmotic pumps are prefilled with 200 µg or 500 µg (or other amount) of the SAg in a total volume of 200 µL of PBS. Miniosmotic pumps are loaded using a 1-cc syringe with a flat-tip needle supplied with the miniosmotic pump kit (*see* **Note 1**).

2. American Dutch belted rabbits are anesthetized with intramuscular (IM) injection of ketamine (40–90 mg/kg IM) and xylazine (3–5 mg/kg IM). For a 1–2 kg rabbit we typically mix 0.5 mL of xylazine (20 mg/mL) and 0.5 mL of ketamine (100 mg/mL) in a ster-

ile syringe and inject IM using a 27-gauge needle.

3. After rabbits are fully sedated, rabbits are shaved on the left flank and a small incision (1.5 cm) is made with a sterile surgeon's blade to the subcutaneous layer.
4. Miniosmotic pumps are implanted subcutaneously.
5. The incision is closed with sutures.
6. Rabbits are monitored for signs of STSS, and mortality (or conditions necessary for premature termination) is recorded over a 15-d period.

3.4. Emesis

We use a standard monkey feeding assay *(15)* with modifications *(16)* to eliminate the need to anesthetize or intubate the animal. These modifications prevent inaccurate results from the emetic action of some anesthetics and accidental administration of the toxin to the lungs by improperly inserted nasogastric tubes.

1. Animals used in the experiments should be trained daily to accept flavored fruit punch from a syringe for a period of approx 2 wk prior to the experiments.
2. On the day of the experiment, the toxin being analyzed should be dissolved in the fruit punch (usually 5 mL) at the desired dose and loaded into a syringe.
3. The fruit punch containing the toxin is fed to the monkeys using the same method with which they were trained (*see* **Note 2**).
4. Once the toxin is administered, the animals should be observed for 8–10 h to determine if they exhibit an emetic response. If desired, the reactions of the animals can be monitored by video recording, provided that routine checks are made so that veterinary care can be provided if needed.

4. Notes

1. For the miniosmotic pump model of TSS, we generally administer either 200 or 500 µg of SAg per miniosmotic pump. For TSST-1, 100–200 µg per rabbit is typically an LD_{100}. For SPE A or SPE C, 200–500 µg per rabbit is typically an LD_{100}.
2. The minimal emetic dose for a typical staphylococcal enterotoxin such as SEC1 in this assay is 0.1–1.0 µg/kg.

Acknowledgments

This work was supported by USPHS grants HL36611 and AI22159 from NIH to Patrick M. Schlievert, and USPHS grants P20RR15587 and R01AI28401, USDA NRI grant 99-35201-8581 and the Idaho agricultural experiment station to Gregory A. Bohach.

References

1. Marrack, P. and Kappler, J. (1990) The staphylococcal enterotoxins and their relatives. *Science* **248,** 705–711.
2. Li, H., Llera, A., Malchiodi, E. L., and Mariuzza, R. A. (1999) The structural basis of T cell activation by superantigens. *Annu. Rev. Immunol.* **17,** 435–466.
3. Kotb, M. (1995) Bacterial pyrogenic exotoxins as superantigens. *Clin. Microbiol. Rev.* **8,** 411–426.
4. Dinges, M. M., Orwin, P. M., and Schlievert, P. M. (2000) Exotoxins of *Staphylococcus aureus*. *Clin. Microbiol. Rev.* **13,** 16–34.
5. McCormick, J. K., Yarwood, J. M., and Schlievert, P. M. (2001) Bacterial superantigens and toxic shock syndrome: an update. *Ann. Rev. Microbiol.* **55,** 77–104.
6. Dinges, M. M., Jessurun, J., and Schlievert, P. M. (1998) Comparisons of mouse and rabbit models of toxic shock syndrome. *Intl. Congr. Symp. Series* **229,** 167–168.
7. Miethke, T., Wahl, C., Heeg, K., Echtenacher, B., Krammer, P. H., and Wagner, H. (1992) T cell-mediated lethal shock triggered in mice by the superantigen staphylococcal enterotoxin B: critical role of tumor necrosis factor. *J. Exp. Med.* **175,** 91–98.
8. Leist, M., Gantner, F., Bohlinger, I., Germann, P. G., Tiegs, G., and Wendel, A. (1994) Murine hepatocyte apoptosis induced in vitro and in vivo by TNF-alpha requires transcriptional arrest. *J. Immunol.* **153,** 1778–1788.
9. Nagaki, M., Muto, Y., Ohnishi, H., Yasuda, S., Sano, K., Naito, T., et al. (1994) Hepatic injury and lethal shock in galactosamine-sensitized mice induced by the superantigen staphylococcal enterotoxin B. *Gastroenterology* **106,** 450–458.
10. Parsonnet, J., Gillis, Z. A., Richter, A. G., and Pier, G. B. (1987) A rabbit model of toxic shock syndrome that uses a constant, subcuta-

neous infusion of toxic shock syndrome toxin 1. *Infect. Immun.* **55,** 1070–1076.

11. Westphal, O., Luderitz, O., and Bister, F. (1952) Uber die extraktion von bacterien mit phenol-wasser. *Z. Naturforsch.* **78,** 148–155.

12. Shnyra, A., Luchi, M., and Morrison, D. C. (2000) Preparation of endotoxin from pathogenic gram-negative bacteria, in *Methods in Molecular Medicine: Septic Shock* (Evans, T. J. ed.), Humana Press, Totowa, NJ, pp. 13–25.

13. Kim, Y. B. and Watson, D. W. (1970) A purified group A streptococcal pyrogenic exotoxin. Physiochemical and biological properties including the enhancement of susceptibility to endotoxin lethal shock. *J. Exp. Med.* **131,** 611–622.

14. Schlievert, P. M. (1982) Enhancement of host susceptibility to lethal endotoxin shock by staphylococcal pyrogenic exotoxin type C. *Infect. Immun.* **36,** 123–128.

15. Bergdoll, M. S. (1988) Monkey feeding test for staphylococcal enterotoxin. *Methods Enzymol.* **165,** 324–333.

16. Schlievert, P. M., Jablonski, L. M., Roggiani, M., Sadler, I., Callantine, S., Mitchell, D. T., et al. (2000) Pyrogenic toxin superantigen site specificity in toxic shock syndrome and food poisoning in animals. *Infect. Immun.* **68,** 3630–3634.

Index

A

Accessory cells, 115, 117
Accessory molecules, 114, 117
Activation marker for T cell,
    186–187, *see also* CD69
Adhesion slide, 175, 179, 181
Animal model for toxic shock
    syndrome, 17–18, 246,
    248–251
Antigen-presenting cell (APC), 1–2,
    18, 101, 113–114, 127, 186,
    188, 190, 205
  APC-responder ratio, 133,
    205–208, 211–212, 215
Anti-CD3, 128–129, 202–203, 205
  crosslink, 190
Anti-inflammatory compounds, 138,
    157–158
Autoimmunity, 16–17, 220

B

Background reduction, 17, 133–134,
    147–148, 163, 166, 171, 179,
    188, 195, 206–207, 211–212
Bacterial superantigens, 1–3, 33–34,
    137–138, 185–186, 245–246
  biologic effects
    anti-tumor treatment,19–20
    disease association, 13–17,
        220, 245
    enteric effects, 219–221
    emesis, 4, 15–16, 246, 251
    in vivo effects, 13, 245–246,
        251

in vivo models 17–18, 246,
    248–251
    pyrogenicity, 33–34, 246,
        248–249
    superantigenicity, 1, 15–16, 246
  blocking peptides, 21
  classification, 2–3, 33–34
  trimolecular complex, 12–13,
        66–67, 70, 77–80, 87–88
  therapeutics against
    superantigens, 20–22, *see*
        also Inhibitors of cytokines
  vaccines, 20–21
  structural characteristics
    3 D structure, 3–4, 56
    binding rate constants, 80
    MHC class II binding, 1, 6–9,
        56, 65–67, 78
    mutational analysis, 7, 9–12,
        20–21
    sequence homology, 3
    T-cell receptor V_β binding, 1,
        10–12, 20, 65–67, 78,
        92–93, 101–102, 106
    zinc binding sites, 7–10, 56,
        65–67
BIAcore^{TM}, 66, 68
    immobilization of protein for,
        71–72
    instrumentation, 68
    kinetic rate constants, 78
Bioassays, 210, *see also* T-cell
        proliferation
Biotinylation, 105

255

C

CD69, 186–187, 193–201, 210–211
Cell fixation, 117, 165–166, 172,
    189, 199
Cell lines
    CaCo-2, 237–238
    CH1(H-2^K) B lymphoma, 67
    CHIE/S7, 49, 52
    CTLL-2, 192
    HT-2, 192, 215
    HT29, 237–238
    Jurkat, 130–131, 134, 222, 227
    Kit, 225, 192
    Raji, 130–131
    T84, 221–223, 236–238, 240
    THP-1, 222, 227
Cell lysis, 131
Cell permeabilization, 165–166
Cell stimulation, 205–207,
    207–208
Circular dichroism, 56, 59–61
Cloning superantigen genes, 36–37
Co-culture of epithelial-immune
    cells, 228–229
Complement-mediated lysis, 116, 124
Contaminants of SPEA, 5
Contaminants of SPEB, 34
Conditioned medium, 228–229
Costimulatory molecules, 113–114
Cytokines, 13–15, 137–138, 151,
    165, 188, 220, 236
    antibodies to, 176–177
    intracellular detection, 166–171,
        175–182
Cytokine assays, 137–138, 141–144,
    191–192, 209–210
Cytokine mRNA, 153–155
Cytotoxicity, 18

D

Denaturation
    chemical, 56, 59–61
    thermal, 56–57
Detection of superantigens, 5–6,
    40–41
Double immunodiffusion, 5, 41

E

Endotoxin, 17–18, 249–250
Enterotoxins, _see_ Bacterial
    superantigens
Emetic activity, 4, 15–16, 18, 251
Epithelial barrier, 14–15
Epithelial cell, 14, 18, 220–222
    co-culture of , 228–229
    ion transport, 230–236
    small molecule flux, 234–236
    transepithelial resistance,
        230–236
Enzyme-linked immunosorbent
    assay (ELISA), _see also_
    cytokine assays
    superantigen binding to TCR,
        106–108
    TCRV$_\beta$ measurement, 105–106
Erythrocyte lysis, 47, 49
Erythrogenic toxins, 33, _see also_
    Bacterial superantigens,
    Streptococcal pyrogenic
    exotoxins
Experimental allergic
    encephalomyelitis, 17

F

Flow cytometry
    application , 49–51, 92–95,
        124–125, 199–200
    cell sorting, 203–205

data analysis, 200–201
detection of viral superantigen,
   49–51
sample preparation, 195–199
Food poisoning, 15–16
FPLC, 68–70

G

Gel electrophoresis, *see* SDS gel
   electrophoresis
Gut mucosa, 219–221

H

HLA-DR, 6–7, 9

I

Inhibitors of cytokines, 138, 157–
   158
Immunoblot, 132–133
Immunoenzymatic staining of cells,
   166–171, 179–180
Immunofluorescent staining of cells,
   166–171, 175–179, 196–199
Immunoprecipitation, 132
Inflammatory cytokines, 137–138
Interferon gamma (IFNγ), 137–138
   ELISA, 143–144
Interleukins, *see* Cytokines,
   Interleukin 2
Interleukin 2 (IL-2), 13, 15, 188
   bioassay, 210
   ELISA, 209
Intracellular cytokine detection,
   166–171
Ion exchange chromatography, 36,
   58
Ion transport, 5, 230–231
Isoelectrofocusing (IEF), 35, 37–38,
   62

L

Lamina propria mononuclear cells,
   225–227
Laser-scanning cytometry, 169–172,
   174
Lymphocytes, 13, 16, 19

M

Mediators, *see* cytokines
Miniosmotic pump, 247, 250–251
Monocytes, 13, 137
   as antigen-presenting cell, 1,
      119–124
   depletion, 226
   fixation, 117
   preparation, 116–117, 124–125,
      226–227, 237, 239
   purity analysis, 124–125
Mononuclear cells, *see* Peripheral
   blood mononuclear cells
Mouse lymphocytes isolation, 193
Mouse Mammary Tumor Viruses
   (MMTV) superantigens, 45–46,
      186
   detection, 49–51
   expression, 49

N

Nickel column, 35, 39

O

Ouchterlony, *see* double
   immunidiffusion

P

Peripheral blood mononuclear cell
   (PBMC), 18
   cell culture, 140–141, 193
   preparation, 140, 223–227
Permeabilization of cells, 165–166, 181

Phage display, 88
Proinflammatory cytokines, 13,
  137–138
Protein A, 19, 132, 134, 190, 214
Protein aggregates, 69–70, 106
Purification of SE, 5
Purification of SPE, 36–40
Pyrogenic toxins, 33, 245–246, *see
  also* Bacterial superantigens
Pyrogenicity measurement, 248–249

R

Receptor clustering, 12–13
RNA
  gel electrophoresis, 157
  probe synthesis, 155
  probe purification, 155–156
  preparation, 153–154
RNase protection assay (RPA),
  154–158

S

SDS gel electrophoresis, 38–40,
  131–132
Shock, *see* Toxic shock syndrome
Signal transduction pathway, 12
Soluble TCR, 67, 102, 106
  Biotinylation, 105
  ELISA, 105–106
  Expression, 104–105
  Isolation and purification, 105
Staphylococcus aureus, 33, 245
Staphylococcal enterotoxins, 2–5,
  137–138, 220–221, 245–246,
  see also Bacterial
  superantigens
staphylococcal enterotoxin A
  (SEA), 55–56, 66–67
  in vivo effects, 15–16, 19–21
  structure, 3–12

staphylococcal enterotoxin B
  (SEB), 55–56, 151–152,
  187, 220–221
  in vitro effects, 152, 157–159,
  234–237, 229–232
  in vivo effects, 15–17, 19–22
  pyrogenicity, 248
  structure, 3–12
Staphylococcal superantigens, *see*
  Bacterial superantigens
Staphylococcal toxic shock
  syndrome, *see* Toxic shock
  syndrome, Toxic shock
  syndrome toxin-1 (TSST-1)
Streptococcus pyogenes, 34–35, 245
Streptococcal pyrogenic exotoxins
  (SPE), 2–10, 33–34, 245–246,
  see also Bacterial
  superantigens
  streptococcal pyrogenic exotoxin
    A (SPEA)
  contaminants, 5, 34
  toxic shock, 14, 250–251
  purification, 5, 36–40
  pyrogenicity, 246, 248–249
  structure, 2–6
  zinc binding, 8–9
  streptococcal pyrogenic exotoxin
    B (SPEB), 34
  streptococcal pyrogenic exotoxin
    C (SPEC), 2–4, 6, 9–12,
    245–246
  streptococcal pyrogenic exotoxin
    J (SPEJ), 3, 33–34, 245–246
  purification, 36–41
Streptococcal superantigens, *see*
  Bacterial superantigens,
Surface plasmon resonance, 66,
  70–77

binding kinetics analysis, 72–80
data analysis,
kinetic rate constant, 78–80
MHC class II binding, 67
Superantigen-induced shock, 13–14,
see also Toxic shock syndrome
Superantigens, 185–186, 220 *see
also* Bacterial superantigens,
MMTV superantigens, Viral
superantigens

T

T cell
activation, 12–13, 34, 45, 127–128,
131, 185–187, 195–201, 211,
220
activation marker, 186–187, 211
preparation, 115–116, 124,
226–227
T-cell hydridoma, 187–188, 200–208,
213–214
T-cell mitogens 189, 212
T-cell proliferation, 13, 15
assay, 117–123, 144–145
data analysis, 123–124
T-cell receptor (TCR), *see also*
Soluble TCR
mutated libraries, 19–21
receptor clustering, 12
structure, 101–102
TCRV$_\beta$ antibody, 189, 197–200
TCRV$_\beta$ specificity determination, 19
Ternary complex, 12–13, 87–88,
101–102, *see also* Bacterial
superantigens trimolecular
complex

Toxic shock syndrome, 13–15, 17,
220, 245–246
endotoxin enhancement, 249–251
Toxic shock syndrome toxin-1
(TSST-1), 2–3, 13–15, 17–18,
220 *see also* Bacterial
superantigens
in vitro effects, 18, 137–138
in vivo effects, 13–15, 17–18, 220
MHC class II binding, 6–9
purification, 5
structure, 3–4
TCRV$_\beta$ binding, 12
Transepithelial resistance, 229–236
Transwell, 224, 228–229, 237 *see
also* Ussing chamber
Tumor necrosis factor alpha
(TNFα), 137–138
ELISA, 141–142
Tyrosine phosphorylation, 128, 133

U

Ussing chamber, 223, 230–233,
239–240
UV spectrophotometry, 56–59

V

Viral superantigens, 3, 45–46,
185–186, 214–215
detection, 46–47, 49–51
stimulation of cells, 195, 207–208

W

Western blot, 132–133

Y

Yeast surface display, 88, 90–92, 96